The Aerobie® Book

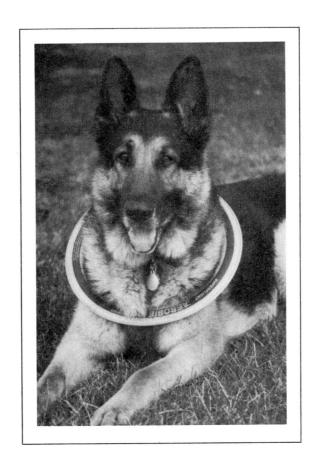

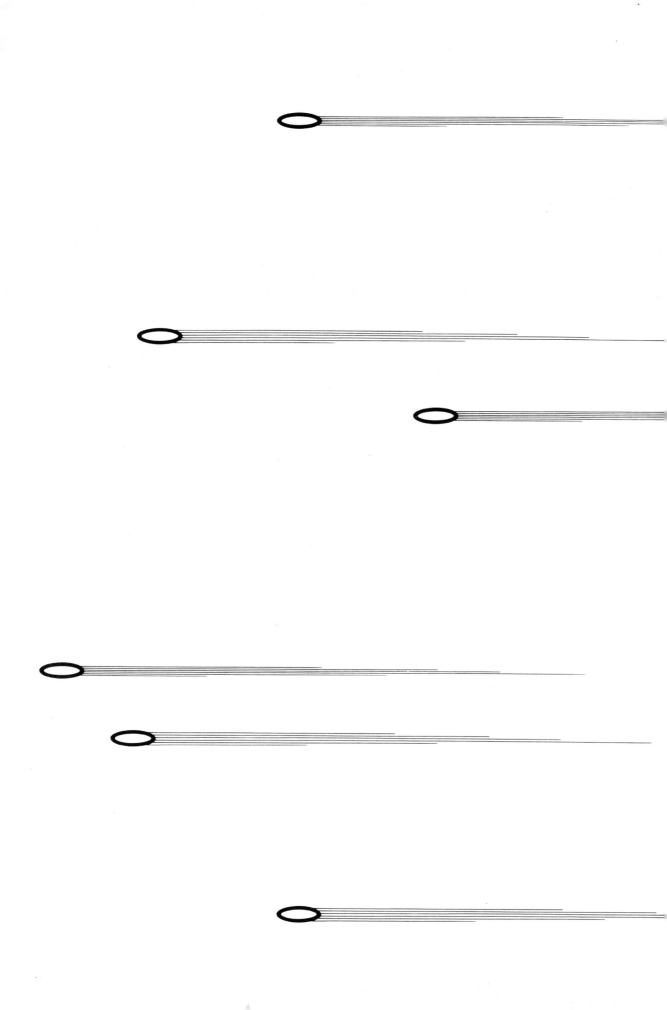

The Aerobie Book

An Inquiry into the World's ULTIMATE Flying Mini-Machine

by John Cassidy

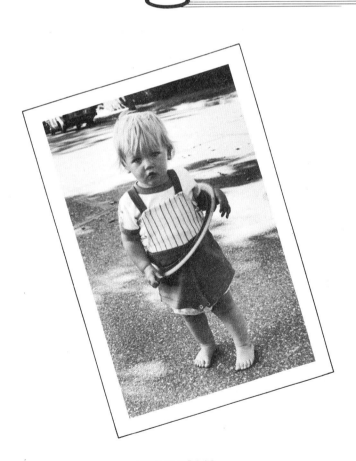

KLUTZ®

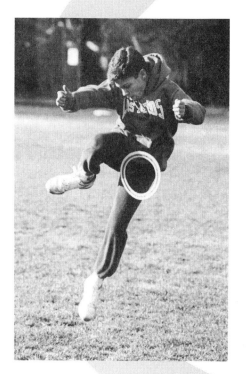

AEROBIE® is a registered trademark for a flying ring toy, manufactured by Superflight, Inc., U.S.A. In this book, use of the trademark AEROBIE® is intended to refer to the AEROBIE® brand flying ring, although for reasons of readability the trademark symbol does not always appear. Activities described in the following text are meant to be performed with the AEROBIE® brand flying ring.

Frisbee® is a registered trademark of Wham-O Mfg. Co., San Gabriel, California, under U.S. Trademark Registration No. 679,186 issued May 26, 1959 for goods specified as toy flying saucers for toy games.

The term Frisbee as used in the text of this book refers solely to the flying saucers manufactured and sold by Wham-O under the trademark FRISBEE® The first letter of the word Frisbee has been capitalized throughout the book as the method chosen to signify that this is a registered trademark.

Design and production by MaryEllen Podgorski and Suzanne Gooding.

Klutz Press is an independent publisher located in Palo Alto, California and staffed entirely by real humans. We would love to hear your comments regarding this or any of our books.

Additional Copies:

For the location of your nearest Klutz retailers, call (415) 857-0888. If they should all be regrettably out of stock, the entire library of Klutz books, as well as a variety of other things we happen to like, are available in our mail order catalogue. See back pages for ordering information.

4 1 5 8 5 7

ISBN 0-932592-30-9

Published by **KLUTZ** ®

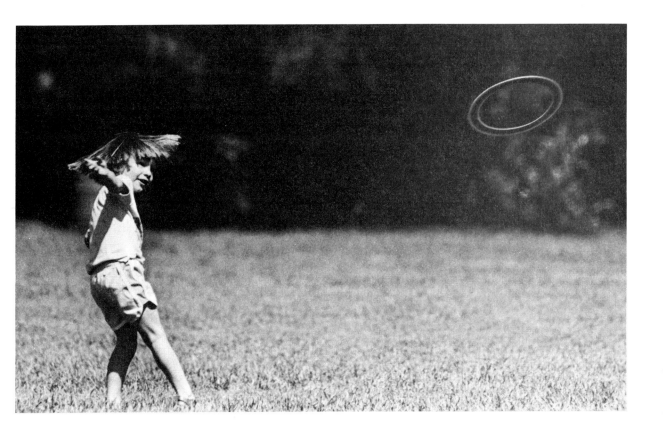

If you stop to think about it, there is hardly anything more basic to the human condition than an irrepressible interest in throwing things. Originally it probably started in connection with the Cro-Magnon problem of being one of the slowest animals on the block, but it soon took on an additional dimension—it was fun. You could turn it into a game. "Catch," in fact, may well be Man's First Game, forming the basis for nearly every other sport ever invented.

And in that sense, this is a book about Basics.

But it's also a book about something quite new, because after some 15 million years, the Aerobie has made the old game suddenly look...very different. You don't have to rear back, hold your breath, close your eyes and aim for the sky anymore. The rules have changed. Gravity's been put on hold. The Aerobie sails. It's like a puck on an invisible sheet of ice. You've never thrown anything more easily, more gracefully, or with more cross-neighborhood range than Alan Adler's amazing new flying machine— the Aerobie.

Welcome to the new game of catch.

Contents

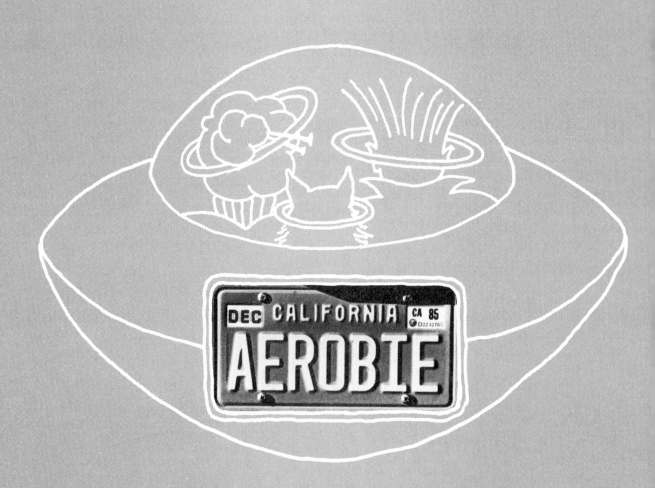

DEC CALIFORNIA CA 85
D2232765
AEROBIE

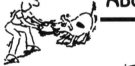
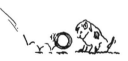

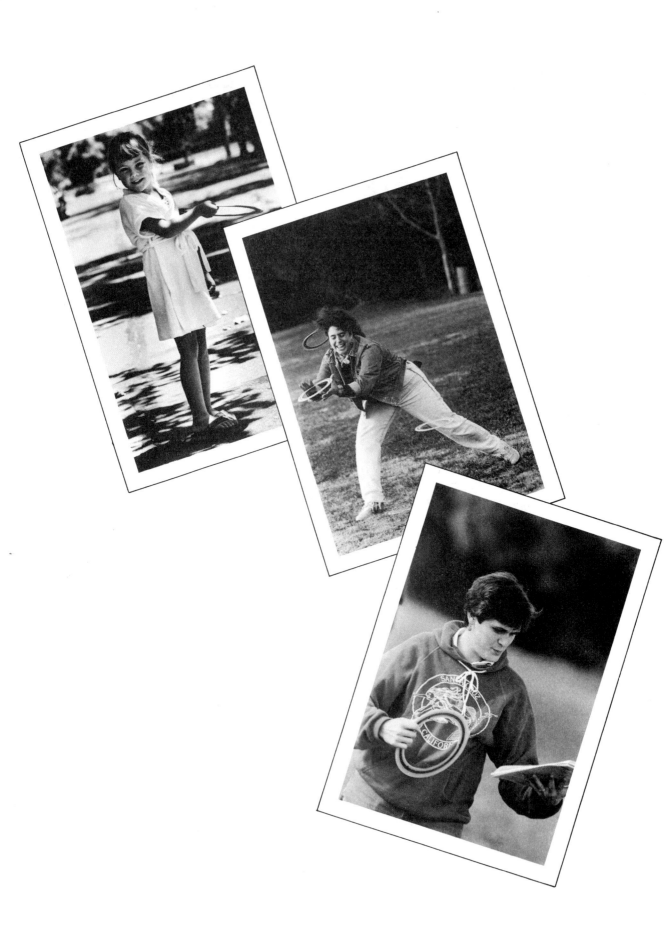

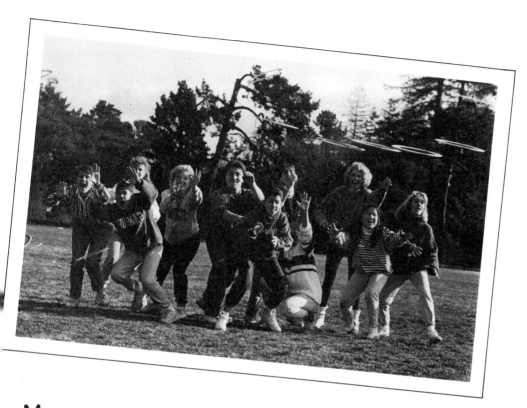

You probably should have read all this first, but by now (let's be realistic) you've long since taken your Aerobie outside and launched it, just to see how it works. After watching it settle into the branches of a tree you thought was well out of range, you've been duly impressed. If you stuck with it some, you may have had problems keeping it flying straight, or getting it to go anywhere near where you were aiming. Chances are it had this tendency to curve off one way or another. And, as you undoubtedly discovered, a little curve at the beginning can put the Aerobie an amazing distance away from anybody by the time it hits the ground. At times, your partner may have felt the need for a bicycle, just to get close.

If you're at this stage, Congratulations! Five minutes into it and you're already playing your first game, called,

Fetch!

For the person doing the throwing, Fetch! can be kind of fun. You get a chance to limber up the arm, test the wind, and really unwind. But occasionally you may have problems finding a partner for Aerobie Fetch! And if that ever happens, you may have to move on to the next step, and the next game.

1

The Standard Sized
Backhand

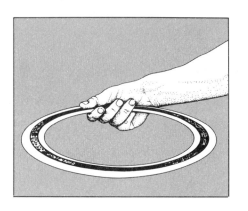

The Long Range Backhand Grip.

This is the basic style, the definitive Aerobie throw. You can spend a contented Aerobie lifetime using nothing but this release.

For medium range (30–90 yard tosses), the key to a straight flight is a dead flat release. And the key to *that* is a stable grip, and a steady, smooth motion. Everyone seems to want to hold on to the Aerobie an instant too long, which tips it a bit and starts a curve in motion. You should snap off a throw. It's almost exactly like popping a towel. You'll add spin to the toss, and in the process, stabilize it.

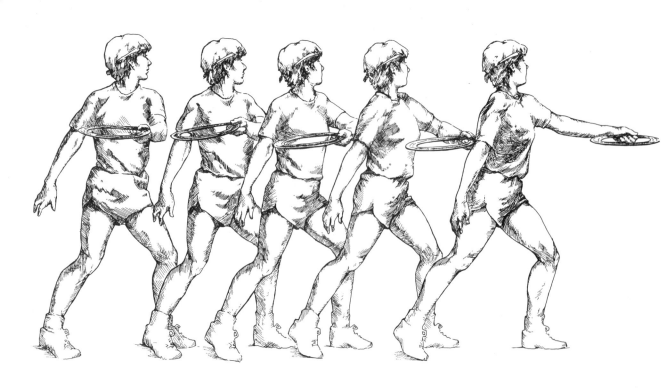

The backswing should be about chest high, even with your release. As you pull the Aerobie back, cock your wrist in preparation for the snap release.

A final note. At this stage, the most common mistake is too much strength. Pull way back on the power and concentrate on being smooth. A perfectly level throw will go an awfully long way without any special effort.

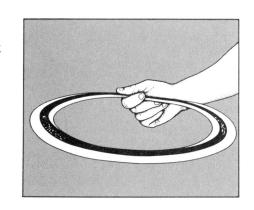

The Short Range Backhand Grip.

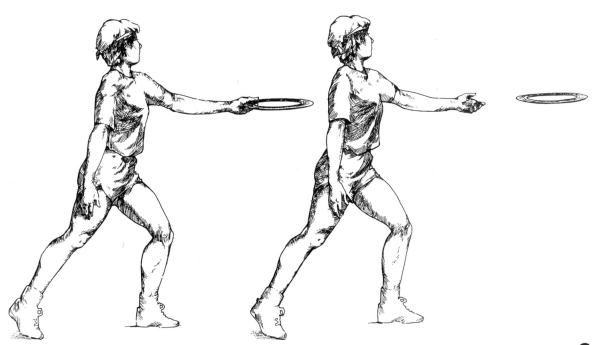

The Standard Sized
Forehand

A trickier throw than the backhand, but still one of the basics. The problem, once again, is the curve. You'll throw the Aerobie, sidearm this time, with a good bit of force because it's the old familiar baseball throw, but it instantly starts to turn radically away from you. Entranced, you and your partner watch as it soars gracefully, over hill and dale, past houses and farms, eventually out of sight.

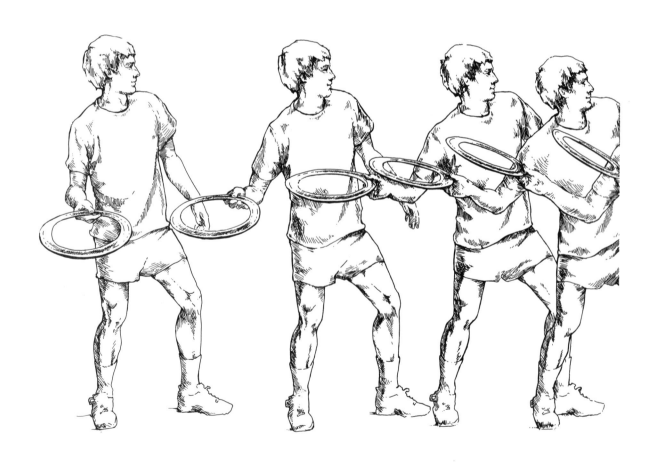

This kind of thing does not encourage repeat experimentation. The solution, once again, is to use less strength. At the risk of repeating myself, you don't need a monstrous throw to get some amazing results with the Aerobie.

The other trick to a decent forearm throw is to over-compensate for the curve by leaning the outside edge (the one away from you) down a tad as you release. If you've got the angle just right, the Aerobie will leave your hand angled *slightly* down, but then flatten out as it flies along. Too much angle, and it'll sail off to the right. Too little, and it'll head off to the left. The determining factor is the strength of your throw.

The tendency, incidentally, is to over-lean it. Angle it down less rather than more, (and don't angle it at all if your throws aren't curving!)

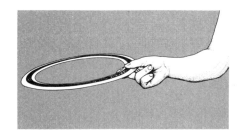

The Forehand Grip. When you release, be thinking "flat."

The forehand is a particularly good release for small-scale front yard kinds of catch and toss games. You can snap this throw off almost entirely with wrist action, hardly any arm at all. Use lots of spin, and remember not to carry your backswing too low or you'll release too high sending the Aerobie to parts unknown.

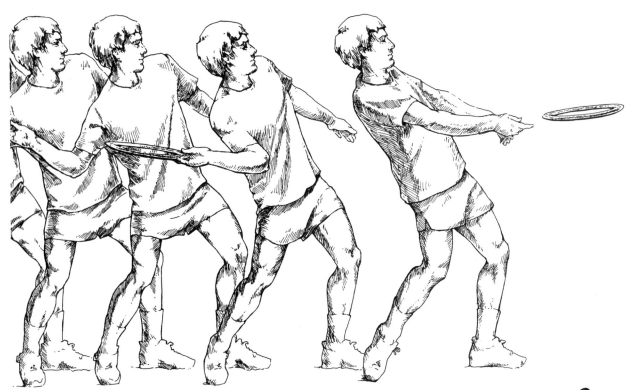

5

The Overhead
Wrist Flip

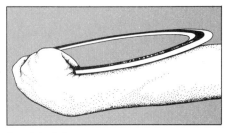

The Flip Grip.

This is the third basic release. It takes a little extra contortioning to keep things flat, but it's really no more difficult than the forehand. Since there's less windup, it's a snappier throw, with lots of wrist action. Keep your elbow nearly as high as your wrist, as per the illustration. And if it helps, lean over from the waist a bit. Incidentally, despite the odd-seeming release, you can put some serious force behind this throw once it's mastered.

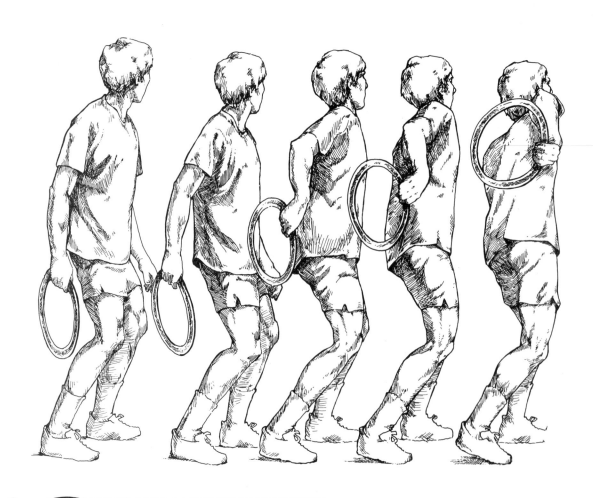

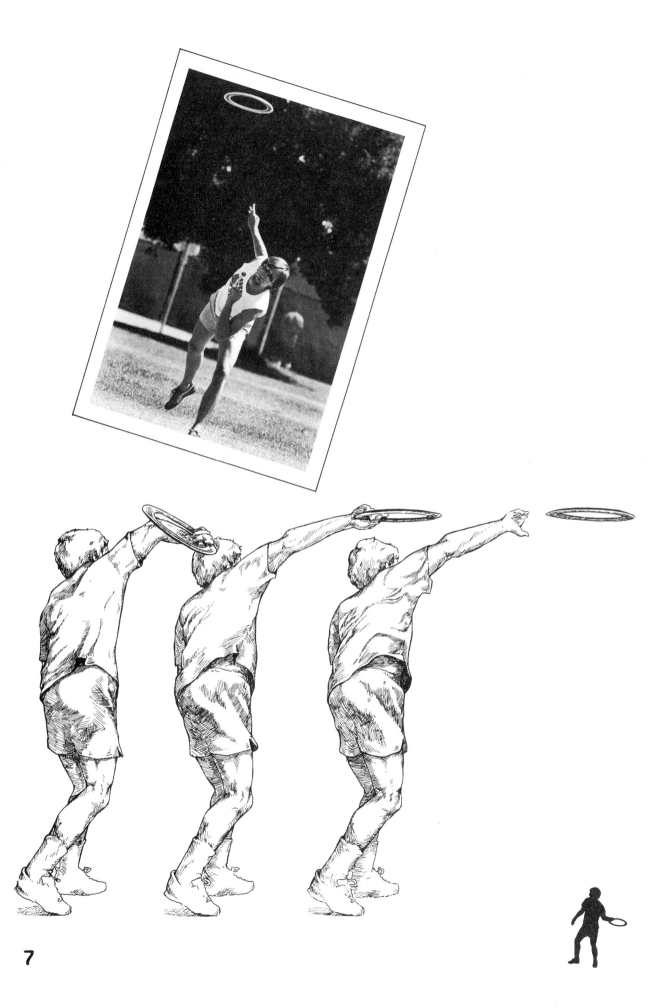

7

Mandatory Reading

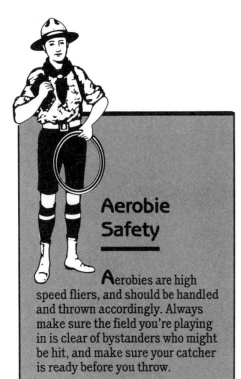

Although it may look sort of low-tech, the Aerobie is actually a very carefully balanced piece of aerodynamic apparatus. Think of it as a small, round Maserati. Incredible performance, but takes a little extra care. And in this case, extra care means

Tuning the Aerobie

The key ingredient to Aerobie maintenance is keeping it in tune. Out of tune, an Aerobie will not fly straight, no matter how incredible your technique.

When an Aerobie leaves the factory, it's checked for balance, but in the process of going from our hands to yours, all sorts of horrible things may have happened to it. As a result, there's a little check-out ritual you should go through the first time you take it out, and in fact every time you go out to throw, since an Aerobie can go out of tune if it's left in a hot car, spindled, bent, folded, or otherwise mauled.

You'll find that after you tune the Aerobie it will have a nagging tendency to creep back toward its prior tune over the course of the next couple of throws. This is normal "sneak-back." Just give it another bend or two as needed. Eventually, your Aerobie will realize you mean business and start behaving.

How to Do It

Back off from your partner 40 or 50 steps, and sail an easy, grandmotherly toss in their direction. To really get the idea, tell your partner to let it go. Don't catch it. By keeping your effort to a minimum, you should be able to release it dead flat. Use the basic Frisbee style flip.

If it leaves your hand absolutely level, and assuming there's no wind, it should maintain that orientation all the way through to the end of its flight. *Right down to the ground.* The Aerobie has been engineered very carefully to yield arrow-straight flights, and you should expect nothing less than perfection.

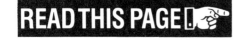

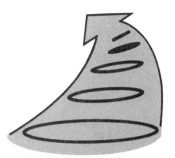

If you're righthanded, throwing with a FLAT standard Frisbee style flip, and it curves left... flex it down.

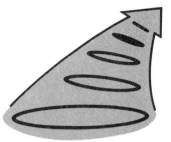

If it curves right... flex it up.

But if you're left-handed, throwing the same way, reverse these directions.

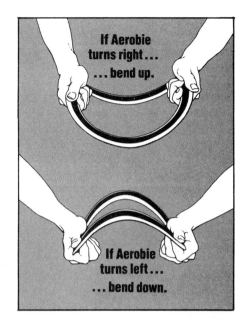

If Aerobie turns right... ... bend up.

If Aerobie turns left... ... bend down.

If it curves, make sure there's no wind, and then try again to see if the problem is consistent. Concentrate on a smooth FLAT release. If your throw is all right, and there's no confounding wind, but it still curves, you have an out-of-tune Aerobie.

If you're righthanded, using a backhand flip, and if it curves to the right, bend it up, with a couple of quick flexing motions. How many depends on the severity of the curve. After a little experience, you'll be able to judge for yourself.

If it curves to the left, bend it down.

If you're lefthanded, a left bearing curve needs upward correction, and a right bearing curve needs downward correction.

Why This Is Important

Just holding the Aerobie in your hands, you won't be able to see the change these corrections will make. The adjustments are too fine. Where they *will* show up though is in the air, where you'll find the Aerobie quite sensitive to this kind of tweaking.

Learning this technique is absolutely critical to your future career in professional Aerobie, and you should learn it well. Ideally, you should find yourself making these corrections automatically. You'll know what a 3-bend curve to the left looks like, and you won't waste any time over-correcting and then having to bend it back. You will also find that this little trick alone will set you apart from the average Aerobie hacker and earn you at least a little respect at the next picnic toss.

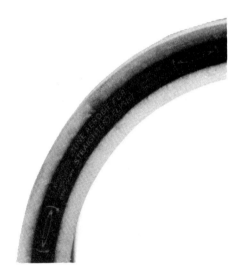

The instructions printed on the Aerobie itself ("If Aerobie turns right, bend up" and "If Aerobie turns left, bend down") are for righthanded, backhand throws. Reverse them if you're a leftie, or throwing forehand.

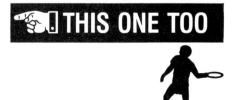

THIS ONE TOO

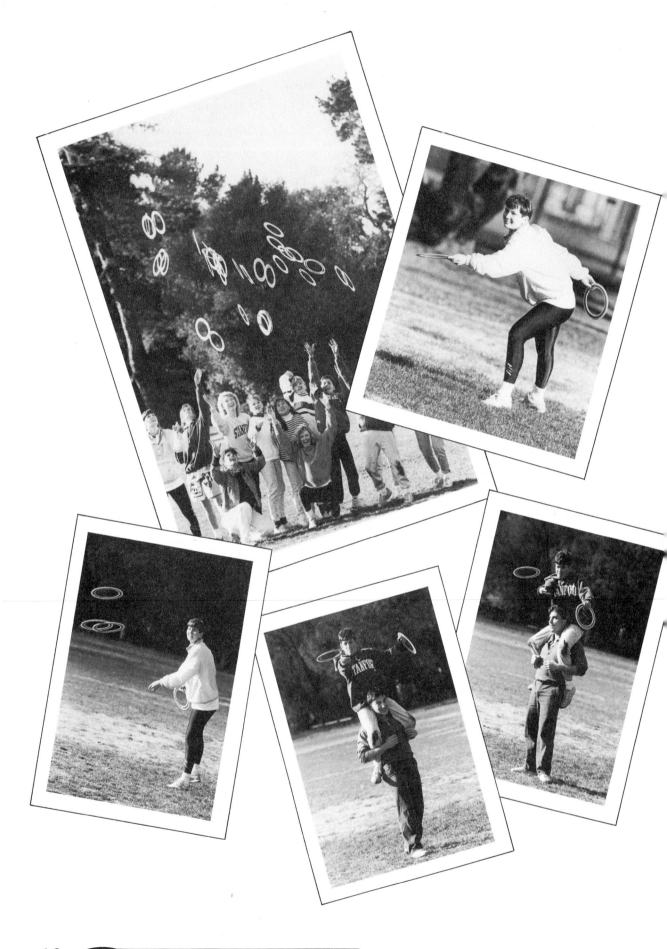

Fancy Tossing

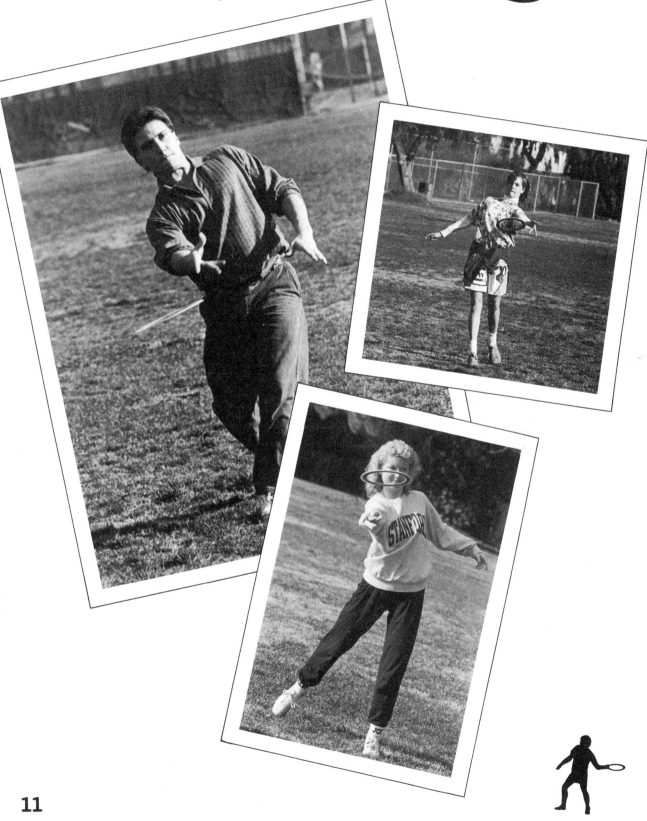

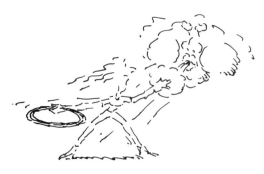

Basic Catches

The big problem here, particularly for the one-handers, is the bounce-out. It comes from the action of the rubber bumper and the flexibility of the plastic backbone.

Probably the best way to minimize the problem is the two-handed sandwich slap. As the Aerobie comes winging by, trap it by clapping your hands together, top and bottom.

If you're dealing with a high thrower that's settling in, the easiest catch is the Aerobie ringer. Just stick your arm through.

If you're too proud to go for anything but the one-handed variations, you might try coming at the Aerobie from the side as it goes whizzing past. All the momentum won't be working against you. Otherwise, just work on developing a good set of mousetrap fingers—and anticipate the rebound.

Dealing with the Wind

Because of the fact that the Aerobie has a thin airfoil, it is quite tolerant of windy conditions, although it still takes a bit of extra finesse.

If you are throwing into light wind conditions, you may have to release your throws with a little extra downward lean to them. But be gentle. Just because you have a headwind doesn't mean you have to pour on the power. Since a headwind will help to keep the thing aloft, an easy toss will carry quite a surprising distance.

Conversely (and contrary to common sense), with a following wind you'll have to give it an extra kick, so that its speed relative to the air stays high enough to keep the Aerobie flying.

If you do much windy flying, you'll find the Aerobie developing a kind of screwball flight pattern. It'll suddenly jump up, then down, then up again. Makes for some exciting receptions.

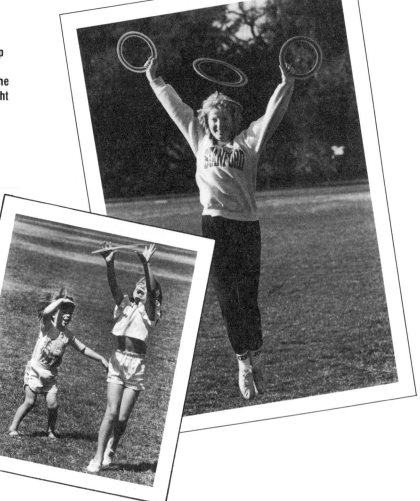

The Not-So-Basic Catches

This is an area for the free-stylers. Once you can make the standard grabs and ringers, you'll undoubtedly start feeling a little cocky. If you aren't careful, you'll soon be going for the behind-the-back, between the legs kind of thing. This is normal, nothing to be worried about, although I would skip the around-the-neck variations.

Tipping the Aerobie straight up, either by hand or by foot, and then catching it on its way down is a freestyle trick that you can sometimes use to good effect if you're going for something either too low or too high. Actually catching it with your foot is a minor milestone on your way to Aerobie greatness.

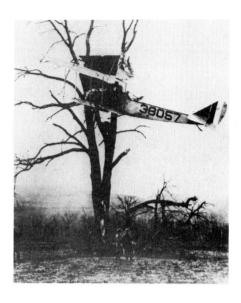

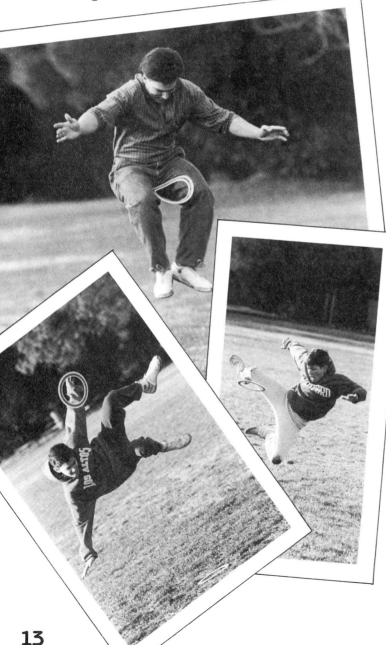

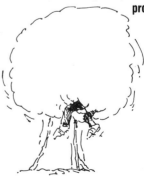

Tree Extraction

By now you have undoubtedly discovered that the Aerobie has a thing about trees. That is to say, it is physically drawn toward them, and once there, it sticks. Passionately.

In a rigorously controlled experiment conducted in Palo Alto, California for example, out of 35 Aerobies deliberately thrown into an average type tree, 26 of them stayed. As of this writing, 3 of them are still there.

Meanwhile, as if that weren't bad enough, they sink like stones. Your first water hazard may well be your last.

In light of these discouraging facts, I would select my playing field appropriately, and bring along a rubber ball just in case. You can use it for attempting to dislodge treed Aerobies.

P.S. I might mention, in passing, a story told by a recent Aerobie tossing business school graduate who climbed a particularly aggressive tree one day in an effort to retrieve an errant throw, and came back with an armload of three Aerobies and 2 kites.

In M.B.A. parlance, this would be described as the upside potential of the tree problem.

The Ten Challenges

In the interests of pushing forward the
boundaries to human achievement
in general, and of Aerobie achievement
in particular, the publisher is hereby
establishing a series of tests to be called
The Ten Challenges. You will find them
described at various places throughout
the text in sidebars.

Throwing for Distance

Everybody's favorite pastime, the
enormous, cross-state, unbelievable-
how-far-can-it-go MONSTER HEAVE.

A word of warning before we get
started on this. Once you get into the
outer limits (150 + yards) accuracy will
start to suffer. This is largely because of the fact that a
very small, normally neglible error (say one degree) at your
release, will yield, when you extend it for 150 yards, some
pretty discouraging results. On top of which, when you
are winding up and putting this kind of force into a throw,
it becomes extremely difficult to fine-tune it for accuracy,
or to keep the nemesis bend out of the flight.

So. Consider yourself warned. And then head for the
nearest open space. Better make it a big one too, a measly
football field won't do. And you better line up a partner
with similar interests and abilities, or you'll be getting your
throws back by return mail, if at all.

Faced with a long throw to make, most people take a
huge breath, tighten every muscle in their body and then
WING it with everything they've got. The results are pretty
unsatisfactory: short, crash-and-burn type flights. At the
risk of sounding a bit mysterious, the trick to avoiding this
problem is only partly physical.

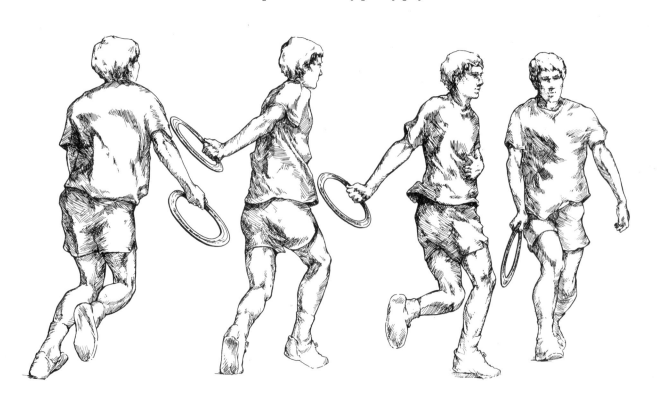

Anyone who has ever spent any time playing tennis, or soccer, or baseball or any number of other ball sports, has undoubtedly had that fleeting, momentary "everything-just-seemed-to-come-together" experience. Suddenly, after what felt to be only a normal effort, you got these incredible results. You took a regular swing, or normal sized kick and then the ball just...TOOK...OFF! It's a wonderfully satisfying experience, frustrating only because you have no way of knowing why it happened, or how you can get it to happen again.

Despite a lot of coaching to the contrary, such moments are hard to duplicate because they represent such inhuman efficiency. For one of those extremely rare instants, we do something with absolutely no wasted motion. On top of which, the end result is perfectly timed and positioned: the ball is hit right on the button, at the precise moment of peak acceleration.

With an Aerobie, the experience is precisely analogous, and you'll recognize it when what felt to be your usual wimpy toss soars way over your partner's head, leaving for parts unknown.

The point of this little digression is to emphasize that it's timing and finesse, not brute strength, that can really make the difference.

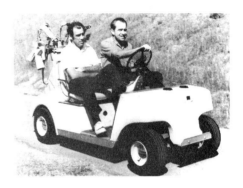
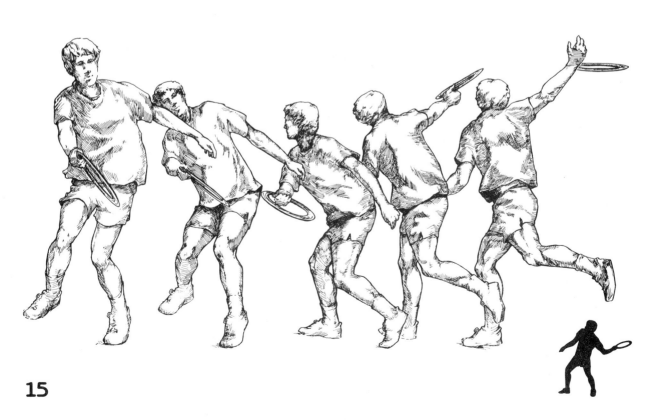

Challenge No. 2
Juggling

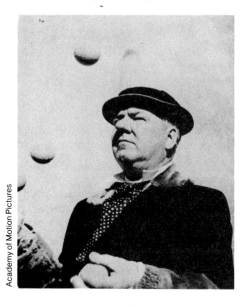

Academy of Motion Pictures

Keep 4 (four) Aerobies cycling between 2 (two) players for a total of 50 throws and catches (25 throws and catches per player). No drops permitted.

Toughness factor: 8

"Yesterday I threw my new AEROBIE into the ocean. The amazing thing was that I was the length of two and one half football fields away from the ocean, and I merely flung the thing ... I wasn't trying for any world records. About twenty people went rushing off to buy AEROBIEs after watching us play."

Shepard Stern
—Marina Del Rey, California

Distance Technique

Look at the illustration for an idea of how to position yourself and your feet. Think of the throwing motion as beginning in your feet, and then building in your legs and torso. Your arm is just the connection between the torque and the Aerobie.

The moment of release should be abrupt, without being stiff. The operative image is "snapping off a throw." All the energy of your throw should leave with the Aerobie.

Try to consciously relax your arm. Think of it as a whip, if it's flexible, the force you put into one end will come magnified out of the other. If it's stiff, half of your effort will be expended in overcoming the "internal resistance."

As I mentioned earlier, with more force in your throw, you'll have to add a little "lean" to the release. The illustration should help, but this is basically a trial-and-error process. The goal is to release the Aerobie at a slight

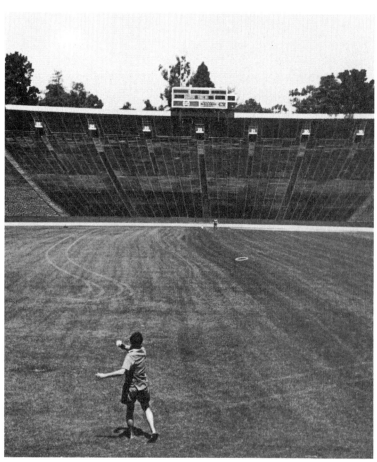

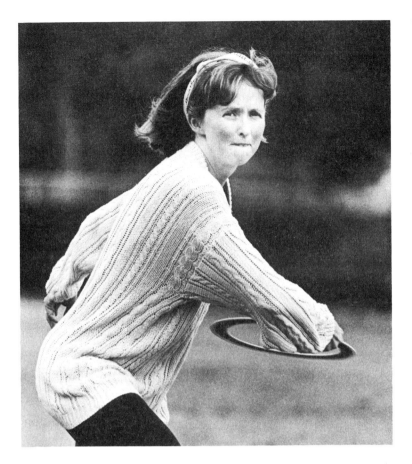

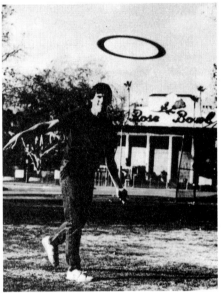

The 1,257-Foot Throw

Scott Zimmerman is an eight-time Overall World Frisbee national champion with an awesome backhand delivery. Standing in the middle of the Pasadena Rose Bowl, Scott can routinely deposit Aerobies, one after another, in the parking lot outside the stadium.

On July 8, 1986, Scott threw an officially measured 1,257 feet, setting a Guinness World Record.

Just to give you some measure of these distances, 1,257 feet is just over 4 football fields, not too much less than a quarter of a mile. Walking, it would take the average person about 10 minutes to retrieve one of these throws.

angle, and then let the force of the throw straighten it out as it goes through the very first part of its flight. Too little lean, and it will curve off opposite to the side you threw it from (to the right if you're a rightie, vice-versa if you're otherwise). Too much lean and it will curve off to the same side as the arm you threw it from. Being able to fine tune this release, with a relaxed arm and a steady grip, is the definition of a good long-distance Aerobie tosser.

In addition, when you're looking for these kinds of distances, you should concentrate on finding just the right height of throw. Angle your throw too high, and it'll waste energy going up and over the top of a parabola. Angle it too low, and it'll hit the ground still with some forward momentum left.

Enough coaching. Take the Aerobie and start throwing. Build up slowly, though. Add strength only to the extent that you can use it. If more strength just stiffens your arm, or causes you to tilt the release, back off until you find a controllable point.

Games

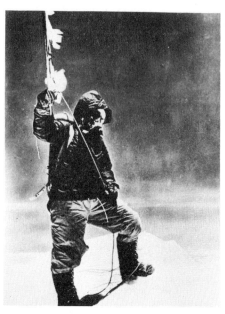

Perfecting a semi-reliable throwing motion, good for throws of 50 to 75 yards, is actually just the First Station in Aerobie mania. Once you've achieved this, you'll soon find yourself looking for additional frustration. It's the human condition.

Enter the world of Aerobie Games.

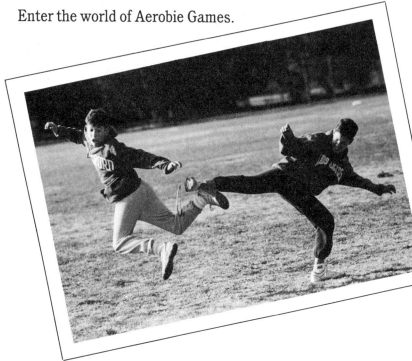

But What Could He Have Done If He'd Had an Aerobie With Him?

High altitude Aerobie throwing is still a newly emerging field, and was unfortunately unknown in 1953 when Hillary and Tenzing first ascended Everest. But, that needn't stop us from a bit of speculation.

The Aerobie has a glide ratio of approximately 10 to 1. It covers, in other words, 10 feet of horizontal as it loses every foot of vertical. With that little fact in mind, we can calculate (very hypothetically) what would have happened if Tenzing or Sir Edmund had sailed an Aerobie off to the Nepali side of the mountain as they stood on the peak.

With a starting elevation of 29,028 feet (and assuming rather uncharacteristically fine flying conditions) such a toss would be capable of traveling just about 55 miles (290,400 feet) if sea level were its final destination. Actually though, the foot of Mt. Everest is not a beach. On the southern flank, Everest rises from a terrain approximately 7,000 feet in elevation. Deducting this from our calculation yields a distance covered of 42 miles. Thus, if the throw managed to clear Nuptse (25,726 feet) to the southeast, that would put its final destination somewhere in the neighborhood of the village of Bhandur, a little less than half the distance back to Kathmandu, or about a 15 day hike from base camp.

Hundred Yard Catch

A game unique to the Aerobie, and accessible to anyone with some motivation, and a fair-to-middling throw.

You'll need a football field. Players stand in either end zone and proceed with your basic game of catch—long distance style. Catches and throws have to be made from within the end-zone. Failure to clear the opposite goal line or stay within the sidelines costs a point. No points are assessed for drops.

Golf

This is a classic game. Simple to play, available to all skill levels, good for any size group.

The immediate inspiration is Frisbee golf. A course is selected, i.e. a school campus, park, city block... one of the best I know of is an abandoned oil storage yard in Jensen, Utah.

Gather together your foursome, designate your first "hole," set par by concensus (*Example:* At the Mt. Rushmore course, the first hole might be Washington's nose. Par 12).

Once everyone has finished the hole, figure how many throws each player was over or under par, and that becomes their score. Then off you troop for the next hole.

A possible variation is to give your caddy both an Aerobie and a Frisbee to carry, using the former as your driver, and the latter as your iron—good for hooks, traps, etc.

> **"I purchased an AEROBIE on March 31, 1986, and since that time, sleep has been difficult!"**
>
> Jody Schaefer
> —Evansville, Indiana

> **"Nothing flies as far, as fast and as fancily as the AEROBIE. It has the speed and distance of the Skyro, the stability of the best Frisbees, and a beauty all its own. It's the logical evolution of the flying disc."**
>
> Dr. Stancil Johnson, M.D.—Author of
> *"Frisbee–A Practitioner's Manual and Definitive Treatise"*

The Front Nine at the Capitol Dome Country Club

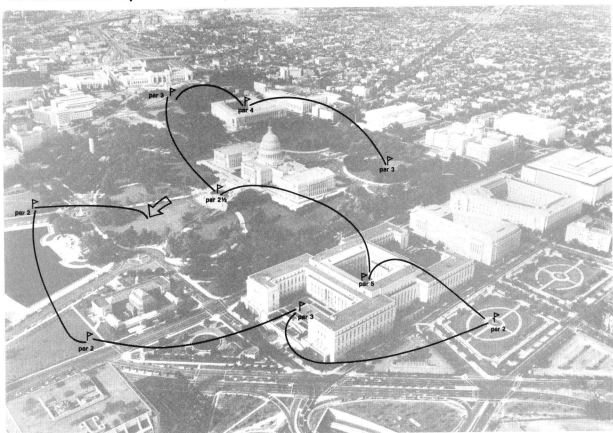

("Where the Servants are Barely Civil")

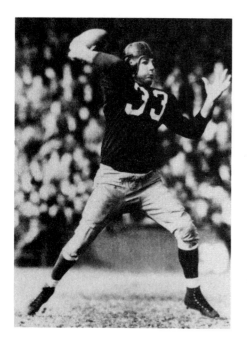

Challenge No. 3
Longest Exchange

Attempt to complete a world record throw-catch-and-return. Only two players allowed. You must complete a throw to another player who must then, immediately and without moving from the point at which he (or she) made the reception, return the throw, which itself has to be caught by the first player. Measure the distance of the shorter of the two throws.

Toughness factor: We'll have to see the record.

Aerobie Argument

A good beginner's game that can be played with any number.

Everybody spreads out, separating by at least 30 yards. Keep the gap between players uniform. The object is to pass the Aerobie from player to player as accurately as possible. If your throw is off the mark, and the catcher has to move in order to make the grab then you (the thrower) are assessed points, one for each step it takes your catcher to get back to his starting point. According to the rules, he has to take uniform giant steps, as big as possible. In practice of course he will try to cheat, taking smaller steps. Efforts to correct this pervasive practice will lead to the confrontations embodied in the name of the game.

Incidentally, if your catcher touches the Aerobie, but then drops it—he picks up a point. If he fails to even *get* to the throw, even though, as any blind man could see, he obviously *could* have, then he also loses a point. On the other hand, if the throw was so lame that there was no way, 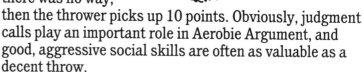 then the thrower picks up 10 points. Obviously, judgment calls play an important role in Aerobie Argument, and good, aggressive social skills are often as valuable as a decent throw.

P.S. First player to 50 loses.

By the Numbers

Cousin to the basketball game of Horse. Best played with two.

The object is to duplicate your opponent's throw and catch. For example: the first player tosses the Aerobie behind his back to his opponent who catches it on his foot. Now the second player has to execute a successful behind-the-back toss to the first player who must then catch it on his foot. Or the first player throws a perfect strike that the second player is able to catch without taking a step. Then the second player is obligated to match the feat. A misplay costs a point. First player to 10 loses.

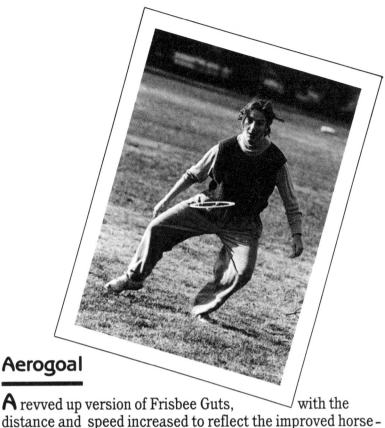

Aerogoal

A revved up version of Frisbee Guts, with the distance and speed increased to reflect the improved horse-power of the Aerobie.

Can be played with any number from one up. The two teams face off at a distance of 30 yards and attempt to throw the Aerobie through (not over, or around) the other team. To be considered fair, the throw must cross the goal line, must be within the sidelines, and must not be over the outstretched arms of the defending team. Throws that are too short, too high, or too wide, are foul and cost the throwing team a point. If a foul throw is caught, incidentally, it's worth 2 points to the receiving team.

And the width of the field is dependent on the number of players. Add 10 yards for every player, and to really liven things up, another Aerobie.

Ten points takes it. Losers buy.

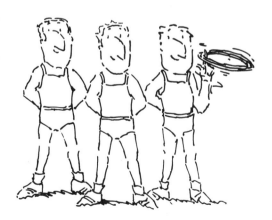

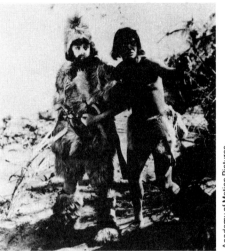

Academy of Motion Pictures

You must cross a significant body of water with a single successfully caught throw. Thrower and catcher must be on different islands, *each of which must have a permanent population and have regularly scheduled ferry service between them.*

Toughness factor: 9

"Thank you for your contribution to the world of fun flying objects ... the AEROBIE is flat-out shocking!"

Tom Bannon—Annandale, Virginia

The History of Flying Flat Things

An Aerobie Pedigree

Challenge No. 5

The George Washington Memorial

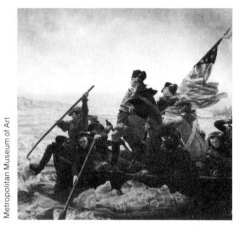

You must complete a double exchange (throw/catch) across the Potomac River, anywhere in the city of Washington, D.C.

Toughness factor: 6

Although it's hard to say exactly who invented the game of catch, records being as vague as they are, one can still speculate as to how the process might have gone. More than likely it was the throwing aspect that came first. At the time throwing was probably a bit of cutting-edge technology spawned by the popularity of hunting fast animals. What was thrown was probably whatever came to hand, and whatever promised to do the most damage when it arrived. Rocks and sticks suggest themselves as the likeliest candidates.

The catching part undoubtedly came later, being a somewhat more civilized activity without the hunting connection. Even if it wasn't particularly valuable from a survival point of view, the discovery that one could actually snatch something out of the air must have made (pre-)history. Again though the objects thrown and caught were probably sticks and rocks, and they may have to count as the world's first sporting goods, just as this prehistoric scenario may have to count as the World's First Game of Catch.

Skipping ahead now some 40,000 years to a modern big league pitcher and catcher, some obvious cultural differences leap to mind between the two settings. But, from a strictly aerodynamic point of view, the ballistics are pretty much identical. Be it a Spaulding Official Major League 132-stitch baseball, or the thigh bone of a small pterodoodaddle, they both conform to the law of gravity in more or less the same way. Up and down. Neither can fly.

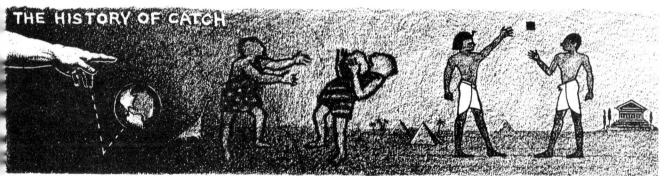

THE HISTORY OF CATCH

THE BEGINNING   1,250,000 B.C.   3,400 B.C.

They can only fall. And how long it takes before they reconnect with the ground is basically a function of the angle and force of take off.

Aboriginal Aviators

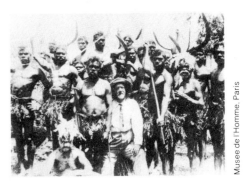

A Group Portrait of Aboriginal Aviators

Pictured above is a collection of boomerang hobbyists taken near the turn of the century somewhere in the Australian outback. It is not at all clear why the hobbyists appear to be so excited, nor is it clear who the disturbed looking fellow in the front is, or if he was ever heard from again.

The historic realization that this apparently inflexible physical law could actually be bent quite a bit if the object in question was appropriately shaped has been most generally attributed to the aboriginals of Australia who began throwing peculiarly carved wooden sticks more than 30,000 years ago. These wooden throwing sticks (or "kylies" in the native tongue) were deliberately carved in the shape of a curved airfoil. It seems a little unlikely that the original owners fully understood the nature of the forces they were tapping into, but it is also quite clear that they knew how to do it.

The sticks were used to hunt small game over the sparsely over-grown outback. While the absence of cover may have made stalking difficult, it was ideal for low-altitude flying. The sticks were thrown, spinning, about rabbit high. The curvature helped them fly straight, and the airfoil, of course, helped them maintain altitude.

While the throwing sticks were the first to make use of the special qualities of the airfoil shape, the true spiritual forefathers of just-for-fun flying apparatus were the *reject* throwing sticks, the ones that were carved so poorly that they had a nasty tendency to curve in flight, some of them so badly that they actually came *back* at the thrower. For a pre-historic family head, having a hard enough time putting kangaroo on the table with a true flying throwing stick, these original boomerangs must have seemed singularly worthless.

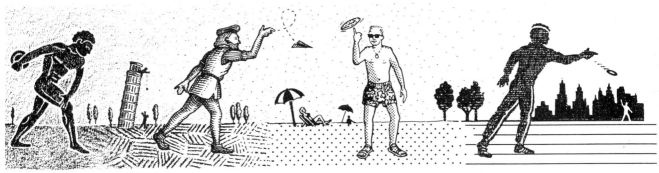

500 BC.   600 A.D.   1955 A.D.   1984 A.D.

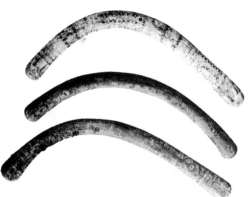

King Tut's Boomerangs

Among the various discoveries uncovered by archeologist Howard Carter in the Tutankhamun find were a number of elaborately carved and decorated boomerangs. The big question, of course, is Sure they look nice, but do they really work?

It turns out this is not such an easy question to answer, owing to the reluctance of some hidebound museum curators who have so far refused any real flight testing, worried that the artifacts would be lost. A feeble objection. Obviously you can't lose a real boomerang by throwing it, and if it doesn't come back, what have you lost? A fake. Thus science is denied.

But they *were* kind of interesting. Plus, of course, difficult to throw away.

Consequently, even in a place and at a time when just staying alive was a full-time pre-occupation, boomerangs were still kept around and, in all likelihood, deliberately carved. Archaeologists have found sport boomerangs reliably dating back to 12,000 B.C. And not just in Australia. Some of the better preserved specimens have been found in Egypt, North America and Europe. Howard Carter discovered a number of elaborately carved and decorated boomerangs in King Tut's tomb.

After these initial breakthroughs in impractical, small-scale aerodynamics, the field appears to have gone into a lengthy period of stagnation. Utility began to rear its ugly head as, increasingly, interest turned toward the bigger scale, with an eye toward possible transportation uses (e.g. the pioneering work of the Greeks Icarus & Son).

Not until Leonardo's groundbreaking work in paper airplane design do we have evidence of some new thinking on the subject of hand-launched aerodynamics. Although, to be honest, Leonardo was actually attempting to address the problems of larger scale flying apparatus by working in miniature. Thus, for the purists, his work is tainted by the suggestion of practicality.

It wasn't until the advent of new lightweight materials (rubber, 1890; pressed metal forms, 1875; stearate plastics, 1933) combining strength and rigidity that the real breakthrough could finally be made, because up to this point, no one had really been walking on the righteous path; the most efficient form remained elusive. The boomerang was an approximation of it, just as the ball was an exaggeration, but there can only be one True Shape of flying things and that is, of course, flat and round.

Joseph P. Frisbie and the Amazing Flying Pie Tin

The year was 1871 and William Russel Frisbie was moving from Branford Connecticut to Bridgeport to manage a new branch of the Olds Baking Company of New Haven. Frisbie was more than just a capable manager though and in a few years had scraped together the necessary funds to buy the bakery himself. He renamed it—for reasons we can only guess at—The Frisbie Pie Company.

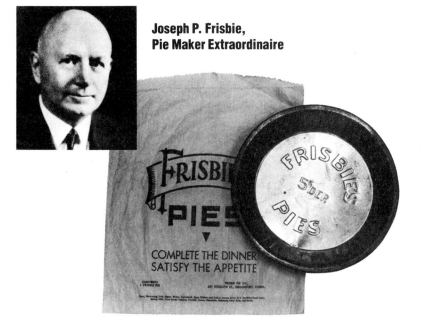

**Joseph P. Frisbie,
Pie Maker Extraordinaire**

An Original Frisbie Pie Tin. Actually not
a bad flier. One was thrown for 62 yards by
Dr. Irv Kalb of New Brunswick, New Jersey
in 1976.

In 1903 W.R. passed away, leaving control of the
establishment to son Joseph P., who oversaw the operation
until his own death in 1940. During his tenure, the Frisbie
Pie Company flourished. Delivery routes were extended.
Shops were opened. Ovens added. It was flush times for
the pie business.

Marian Rose Frisbie, Joseph's widow, carried on ably
after the death of her husband. It was in fact during her
management that production climbed to a new all-time
peak: 80,000 pies per day in 1956!

It was also during this period, the Marian Rose Era,
that the events transpired which ultimately led to such
fateful consequences...

Neither Mrs. Frisbie nor her long-time plant manager,
Joseph Vaughn, remembers the exact year, nor who made
the original breakthrough, but what *is* certain is that at
an early date the decision was made to package the star
product of the company in...PIE TINS! Metal things.
About 10 inches round. Additionally, on the bottom of
these tins would be stamped the words: "Frisbie Pies."

Challenge No. 6
The Headliner

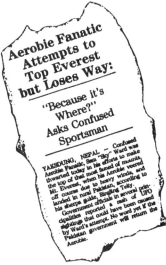

You must concoct some Aerobie
feat interesting or difficult enough to
garner newspaper coverage. (42 days
of continuous throwing...? A ringer
over the top of the Eiffel Tower...?)

Toughness factor: Depends on the size of
the headline.

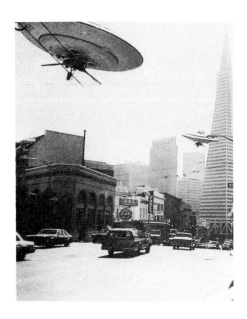

They Came from Outer Space

Flying saucers have been the alien vehicle of choice for as long as extraterrestrials have been making the trip to earth. And with good reason. Rockets lack the all-important ability to hover. Saucers combine great speed with great flexibility. You can stop, look around, do a little laser damage maybe, then suddenly roar off. Not so with a rocket.

When Fred Morrison originally looked to the flying saucer as an inspiration for the motif of his disc, he was actually only returning the favor, since science fiction screenwriters originally settled on the disc shape for its superior aerodynamic performance. It was already a very plausible airborne shape. This is why you can watch so many late movies without seeing a single flying pyramid from outer space.

Once these decisions were made, events followed swiftly, almost inevitably. Customers of the Frisbie Pie Company, once finished with the product, were now faced with a packaging disposal problem. Efforts to solve the problem soon led to a startling aerodynamic discovery, the details of which I will spare you but whose upshot led to a mini-craze in pie tin tossing, particularly on the local college campuses.

This was more or less the state of affairs through the 20's, 30's and 40's, and would perhaps even be the state of affairs today, were it not for Fred Morrison, Walter Francioni and butyl stearates.

Walter Frederick Morrison, a recently discharged GI, had just landed a building inspector's job in Southern California. It was 1948. The country was in the midst of its post-war euphoria—a national case of adolescence—and the mood was ripe for fads. Among the favorites were UFO sightings, invading aliens, and flying saucers.

Like his father, the inventor of the sealed beam head-lamp, Fred Morrison was a tinkerer, an it occurred to him that there might be a way to capitalize on this latest craze. As a youth in Utah, Morrison had flung pie tins and paint can lids around, and now he and his co-worker Francioni began a little informal research into ways one might be able to improve the flight characteristics of these early discs.

Originally, Morrison and Francioni worked in metal, welding rims onto pie tins, but it wasn't long before they began running into the predictable problems. Metal discs were too heavy, too awkward and too dentable. Besides, metal was an Iron Age material, and the two inventors were clearly working in a New Age form.

Enter Polybutyrate Stearates

At the time, plastic was relatively new to the general marketplace, although it had existed in laboratories for more than 20 years. Morrison originally worked in a butyl stearate, a rather brittle formulation that tended to shatter whenever the sun went down. The original model was called Morrison's Flyin' Saucer and by today's standards, not a very good performer, although by changing to a softer polyethylene plastic, they were able to solve the breakage problem.

In 1951, Morrison redesigned the Flyin' Saucer, renamed it the Pluto Platter, and began selling it on the streets and at county fairs. A few years after that, in 1955, he turned over the idea to a start-up company located in San Gabriel, California. Shortly afterward, one of the co-owners, Richard Knerr, was on a trip to the East Coast touting the new product when he began running across students who seemed quite familiar with the idea, only they used the name "Frisbie" and kept looking for something to eat with it. The edibility factor was a bit confusing, but Knerr liked the new word enough to take it with him. Shortly thereafter (in 1957 to be exact), the first plastic disc trademarked (and misspelled) "Frisbee" rolled off a San Gabriel production line that has since produced hundreds of millions.

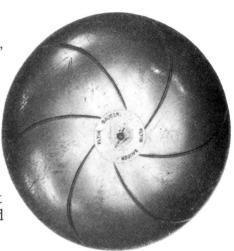

Whether the original makers fully understood the aerodynamic theory of their new invention is a little unclear, but the secret to the straight flying magic of a disc lies in the turbulence created by the thick rim. For reasons that I won't force upon you here, this enables all the lift to focus upon the disc's center of gravity. If it were otherwise, the disc would roll off to one side or another. Unfortunately, a thick rim creates a good bit of resistance as well.

But this seemed a small price to pay for something that flew in such an amazing new way and so, for years, the ancient ball and the new age disc were thought to be the earthbound aerodynamicist's only possible tools.

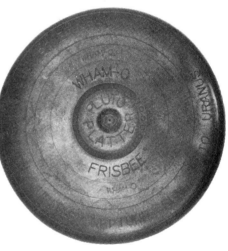

Until 1978.

That was the year that Alan Adler developed his first flying ring, called it the Skyro, and began redefining some of the old terms.

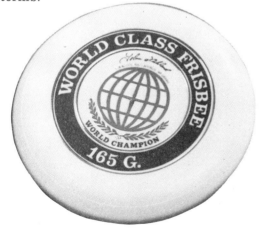

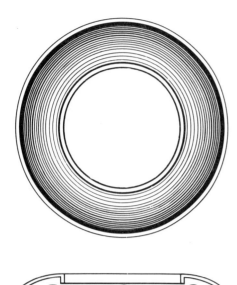

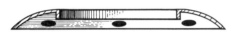

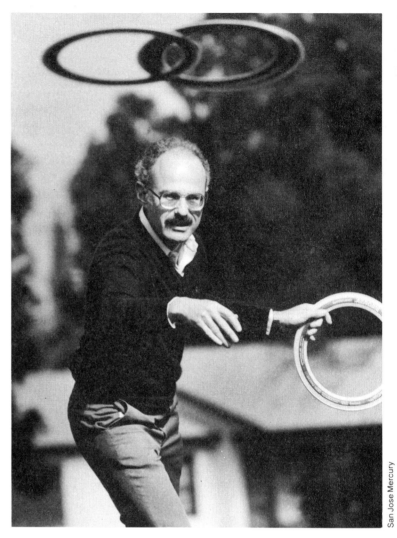

San Jose Mercury

Quoits: The Original Flying Rings?

Anyone searching the patent files under the heading of "rings, flying" would very soon come upon something called "quoits," a game in which the object was to toss a set of rings over an iron stake set into the ground. A little Britannica research would subsequently uncover the fact that quoits has been around since the 16th century, when it was, apparently, quite the rage.

The rings used in quoits were no more than metal doughnuts—fallers, not fliers, fine for the 16th century perhaps, but a bit old-fashioned seeming in the post-Wright brothers era. As a result, in an effort to modernize the sport (and reverse declining fortunes), a number of inventors tried to inject a little aerodynamic flash into the old game by utilizing lightweight materials and adding new features. The ring pictured in the patent application above, for example, could fly through the air while playing a little tune!

It was too little, too late, though. As time went on, quoits lost even more ground to the new more exciting game "horseshoes," and good quoits players could only watch enviously as all the big money and prestige gravitated toward the hot new sport. Eventually, of course, quoits ended up in the dustbin of history, but not before planting the seeds of "ring flight" in the collective unconscious where, years later, they would finally cross-pollinate with flying discs and bear amazing fruit.

Alan Adler

Alan Adler combines a well trained technical mind with your basic schoolboy's sense of invention and fun. In an era of specialization, he is a throwback: an electronic engineer/naval architect/aerodynamicist/computer programmer and freelance intellect. A member of the Stanford engineering faculty, the holder of some 20 high- (and low-) tech patents, the designer of 18-meter racing sailboats and 6-meter racing canoes, Adler combines the skills of an engineer with the spirit of a practical dreamer.

Adler started thinking about long-range hand-launched flying apparatus in the early 70's when he began looking for a technological fix for a distinctly average Frisbee arm. Anyone familiar with aerodynamic principles would have no difficulty recognizing the drag inherent in the basic disc design.

The most obvious solution, driving a truck over the disc to flatten it out, unfortunately yields mediocre results. Even remodeling the disc less abruptly doesn't help. The reason being that drag is a necessary feature to the disc's stability. Without the high drag coefficient, it won't fly straight. Efforts to radically stream-line the design unavoidably de-stabilize it.

After building and eventually discarding dozens of prototypes, Adler hit upon a new approach to the problem. Using a low-profile ring design, he started tinkering with the angle that the ring presented to the on-coming air. Without dragging you through the specifics, stabilizing a flying ring depends on providing both the front and back with an identical degree of lift. Unfortunately, the back of the ring is always flying in the downdraft of the front. Consequently, it normally feels a smaller lifting force than the front, and that throws the ring's balance off.

Crash.

Challenge No. 7
Interstate Transport

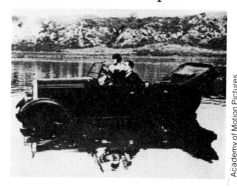

Academy of Motion Pictures

You must throw from one state over a river more than 100 yards wide to your partner who must catch it in another.

Toughness factor: 5–8, depending on your river.

Update on Challenge No. 7

It's been done. Five-time world flying disc freestyle champion Donny Rhodes sailed an interstate Aerobie from Nevada to Arizona across the Colorado River near Laughlin, Nevada on June 10, 1989. Midway across the river, the Aerobie went from area code 702 to 602, while moving from zip code 89029 to 86430.

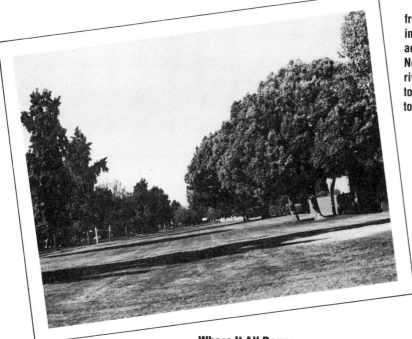

Where It All Began

Pictured above is Alan Adler's Kitty Hawk, the front to the Alza Drug Company on California Avenue in Palo Alto, California. It was here, in 1975, that the first stable ring flew. For Adler, it was the long-sought vindication of years of effort and a magical moment. ("It made my week.")

Also pictured, in the background, is the first Aerobie eating tree.

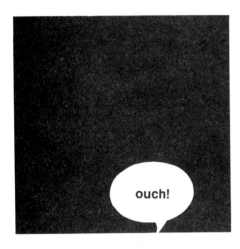

ouch!

You must complete a 150 yard double exchange (throw/catch/throw/catch) in an unlighted field at least 2 hours after sunset.

Toughness factor:
5–8, depending on the moon.

Adler approached the problem by fine tuning the angle that the rings were molded in. The outcome of this experiment was eventually called a Skyro, an extremely low-drag shape that was stable at a specific speed. It was a bit quirky because of this last requirement, but if you learned the tricks to controlling it, the Skyro could be thrown for some unheard-of distances. Standing on home plate, for example, Tom McRann once threw a Skyro clear out of Dodger Stadium, something even Mickey Mantle never managed to do.

Unfortunately, the Skyro's single speed requirement rendered it more or less unstable in the hands of the average thrower, and from Adler's point of view, it was no more than a partial solution to the problem.

Back to the Drawing Board

In the winter of 1984, Adler designed a computer simulation of ring flight. The results indicated that perfect balance (at all speeds) *was* possible, but only if the airfoil could be shaped in such a way that it produced 50% greater lift slope when flying forward than when flying backward. (You know, *lift* slope.)

Anyhow, the *How It Works Section* gets into this in more detail, but this 50% relationship was a good news/bad news piece of information. The good news being that a solution seemed possible. The bad news being that it was all on paper.

Undeterred, Adler plunged ahead with a new series of prototypes trying to meet the 50% requirement. The first 3 all had had the same problem as the Skyro. Good at one speed only.

Then came a breakthrough. The 4th effort was built with a spoiler lip on the outside of the rim. From the very first toss, it was clear this design was going to be different. No matter how you threw it, the spoiler lip kept the ring on an even keel. Adler knew he'd finally hit paydirt.

The final stage was a systematic series of tests to refine the lip and the overall geometry of the outer rim. A dozen models with different heights and angles were made and tested. At the end, one configuration stood out as being the optimal. That shape became the Aerobie.

A mold was designed and ordered in the summer of 1984, and production was finally begun in December. Then on July 8, 1986, Scott Zimmerman threw an Aerobie 1,257 feet, setting a new Guinness World Record for the longest throw in history of any heavier-than-air object.

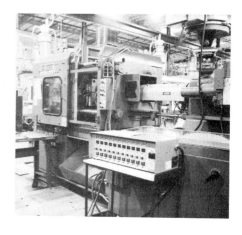

The Aerobie Machine

Aerobies are constructed in a two-step molding process. In the first, the center part (the "armature") is formed. In the second, the rubber bumper is bonded to the armature under more than 1,500 pounds of pressure. The process is a technique unique to Aerobies (and previously, Skyros), which Adler himself developed.

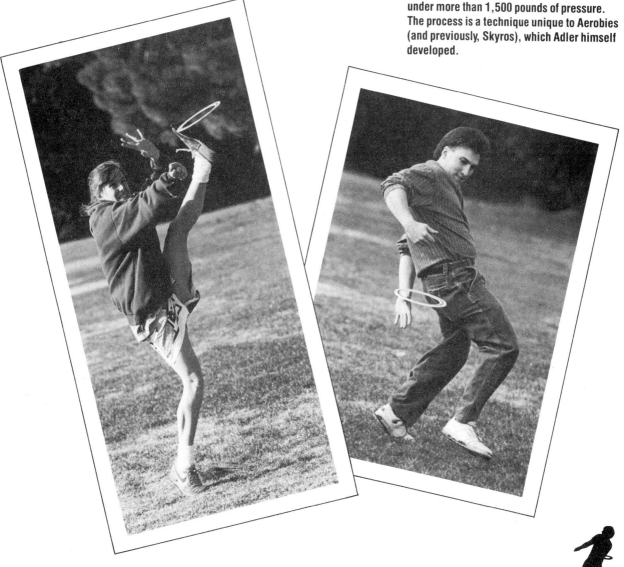

How Works an Aerobie:

The Importance of Air.
The Problem of Gravity.

Daniel Bernoulli was a brilliant 18th century Swiss mathematician with family problems. In particular— his father, who resented his offspring's evident abilities. Johannes I felt as if all of his son's ideas were actually stolen from his own work. It was a family quarrel that all of scientific Europe was kept abreast of via a stream of irate letters and claims that Daniel's father kept publishing.

Every parent has his own final breaking point, a line that he has to draw, and for Johannes I it was *Hydro-dynamic Principia* which Daniel published in 1738. For most people, the book was a rather dry treatment on the subject of fluid behavior under pressure, but for the senior Bernoulli, it was the last straw. Daniel was told to clear out his bedroom and vacate the family premises.

Among observations made in the book, which has since come to be regarded as a piece of inspired research, was one that had to do with pressure exerted by a fluid in motion. The principle it postulated (subsequently named, rather ambiguously from his father's point of view, Bernoulli's Effect) described the relationship between static and dynamic pressure in a fluid, noting that, as the speed of a fluid or gas increased, the barometric pressure of the area it occupied decreased. By installing an airfoil shape (curved on the top and flat on the bottom) in a stream of moving gas, one could create an area of fast moving gas (on top) and an area of slower moving gas (on the bottom). And, as was later observed, this would create a difference in pressure above and below the airfoil, which would, in turn, generate "lift."

If you would feel Bernoulli's Effect at work, stick your hand out of the window of a moving car and angle it slightly upwards. The lifting force that you feel owes much of its existence to the forces Bernoulli described. If you would like to feel even more personally attached to these abstracts, look out the window the next time you're in an airliner. You may have a number of reasons for travelling,

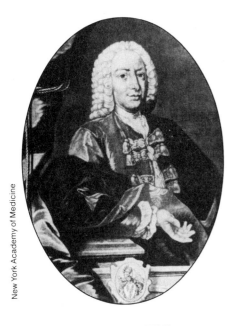

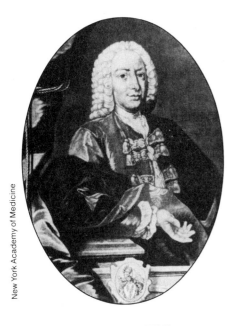New York Academy of Medicine

Daniel Bernoulli (1700–1782)

Daniel was a member of what is generally recognized as one of the most amazing families in the history of mathematics. Starting with Nicolous Senior (1623–1708), and persisting for the next two generations, a total of 9 Bernoulli sons rose to the very forefront of the European scientific community of the era. Three of them, Jacob I, Johannes I and Daniel, made contributions that have secured them a place forever in the history of science.

but Bernoulli's Effect is the only reason you have for staying up in the air.

It is, of course on a much smaller scale, the same principle at work supporting the Aerobie. Gravity is put temporarily at bay by aerodynamic lift.

But the genius of the Aerobie is not so much its aerodynamic efficiency, but the balancing act it performs.

Fun with Flying Cardboard

To get an idea of the problems inherent in balancing a flying disc, conduct the following low-cost research project: Throw a piece of cardboard, angled slightly upward, in the same way you would launch a paper airplane. (In other words, push it straight out, without any spin.) It will almost immediately head straight for the sky. It will not glide along. The reason (trust me) is that the aerodynamic force is concentrated toward the front end. This inclines the cardboard a bit, creating more lift, which again inclines the cardboard creating even more lift, which … In a moment, the cardboard has flipped end-for-end.

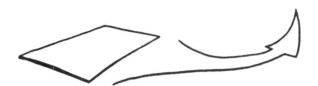

Now, take the same piece of cardboard and (nothing up your sleeve) this time flip it away from you with a spinning motion, Frisbee style. Note carefully the change in behavior. No longer does it try to stand on its tail, now it wants to roll over. Think about this for a second. The cardboard is sailing along, same as before. Bernoulli is right there to deliver the same kind of uppercut to the front end, and yet, instead of kicking up, it rolls over.

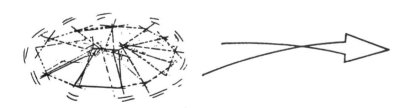

Wherefore the big change?

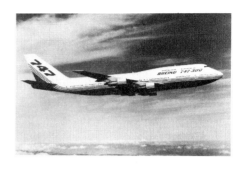

This Is an Amazing Photo

The object pictured above is more than 200 feet long. Three hundred and ten people can sit in it. It shows movies, plays music and serves meals. Sort of. It weighs well over 200 tons, more than an average 4-story building. And it flies.

Figure that one out.

"It's easy to throw. I can control it as well as a Frisbee, but it's more fun because I can throw it farther. It's totally amazing."

Teresa Gaman
Four Time World Frisbee Champion

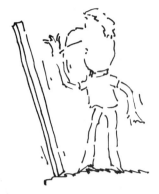

Step 1.

Push on 2 x 4 . Watch as it falls over.

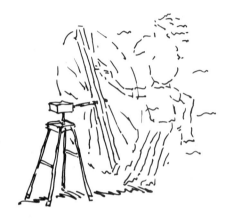

Step 2.

Mount 2 x 4 on bearing. Spin it and push in same place as before.

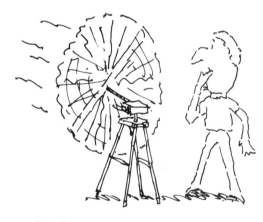

Step 3.

Instead of falling over, it rotates away from you. Confusing, isn't it?

The answer to this, unfortunately, gets a little ugly.

For reasons that I defy you to understand, spinning things react to pushes and shoves sort of peculiarly. I can illustrate this weird behavior with another research project, this one conducted mentally.

The Spinning 2x4 Precessional Research Fantasy

Take your average imaginary 2 x 4 and stand it on its end. Then give it a little shove at its top. What happens? It falls over. Big surprise. Now, supposing you could mount it on some kind of bearing in the middle and then could spin it. So now you're standing in front of a 2 x 4 propeller, whizzing away (you can, in fact, think of it as a wooden "disc"). If you would be so foolish as to try to push near the upper edge of this wooden fan, in the same way as you did before (when it wasn't moving) *it would not fall over.* Instead, the whole right side of this "disc" would turn away from you. It's exactly as if you gave the thing a shove, but on its side, not on the top.

This behavior is called gyroscopic precession, and don't worry, it's not going to be on the quiz. I am told the only real explanation for it is mathematical. If you would like to curl up with the relevant equations, I understand you can find them in Barger & Olson's *Classical Mechanics* (McGraw Hill, 1973). For me, just believing that it even *happens* was bad enough.

Meanwhile, though, back at the original research project.

Since this experimental cardboard flier is spinning when the air lifts it near the leading edge, it *responds* as if it were being lifted, not near the front as any reasonable person would suppose, but near its side (see the confusing two paragraphs above for illumination). The result: the cardboard rolls instead of flipping end-for-end.

From a designer's point of view, whether the ring rolls on its side, or head over heels, it doesn't really matter. Neither is acceptable. The problem is shaping the thing so that the lift focuses itself precisely at the center of gravity. (It's exactly as if you wanted to balance the object on the point of a pencil. Only one place will work).

From our earlier work in unadorned cardboard disc flying, we know that a flat shape doesn't do it. The lift hits it too far forward. By itself, just cutting out the middle of the cardboard doesn't do the job either. Although it's important, it's not *just* the ringification of the Aerobie that makes it stable.

What *does* make the difference is that old familiar concept, downwash angle.

As your average airplane flies forward, its wings cut through the air—re-directing it downward (creating the aforementioned "downwash"). How steeply is described in the term "downwash angle."

Since airplanes rarely fly in reverse, it's the tail of the plane that has to fly in the downwash of the wings rather than vice-versa, but all aircraft have a downwardly pressing tail anyway. It's essential for stable flight, as the unfortunate pilot of the Caproni seaplane too soon discovered (see box below).

A ring designer is up against the same problem. The back half of the ring is always flying in the downwash of the front, and if the associated loss of back-end lift is not corrected for somehow in the design, the result will be instability. The ring will "roll" just as the cardboard did.

In the Skyro, Adler tried a reverse variation on the traditional solution. He *increased* the rear wing angle of attack.

And it worked. The Skyro was stable. But only at one speed.

The problem was the lack of an on-board pilot who could trim the Skyro as it flew along to account for the changes that varying speeds made to the downwash angle. A slow Skyro creates greater downwash than a fast one. And with a fixed set of angles molded into the Skyro's edges, front and rear, there was no room to adjust for these changes. At lower speeds, the Skyro rolled to the left; at higher speeds, to the right.

What was needed was a fixed wing shape (or, in this case, rim shape) that was built in such a way as to compensate for these changing conditions, without having to be changeable itself.

It was a tall order. Starting in about 1979, Adler began tinkering with the equations and built various prototypes, without much success. In 1984, he designed a

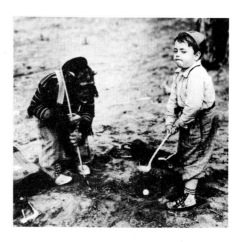

Challenge No. 9
The Handicapper

On a good day, when all the signs are favorable, 160 yards is not an impossible throw for someone with a fair bit of experience in the area of throwing things. Using that as a "par" figure for the age group 16–35, what follows is a handicap table for all those younger or older.

AGE	PAR
2–16	160 minus 10 yards for every year under 16
18–35	160
35 +	160 minus 2 yards for every year over 16

The Challenge then is to score over par for your age group. Note this is *not* a challenge for the group between 18 and 35 and further note that your throw has to be caught in order to count.

If you're younger than 18, or older than 35, and you've managed a throw well over par, send it in. We'll keep two separate classes (men's and women's), and we'll print the best of each.

computer program to simulate the flight conditions and was rewarded with the first solid piece of progress. Theoretically at least, it appeared that such a balanced design was possible. But there had to be a precise relationship between its flight characteristics when the airfoil was at the front of the ring flying "backward," then those occurring half a revolution later when it was at the back flying "forward." The critical issue, the program suggested, was the change in lift for any change in the angle of attack.

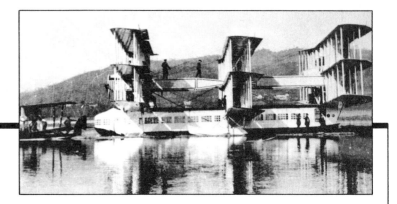

The Seaplane and the Skyro

On the surface, there appear to be a number of important differences between the Skyro and the seaplane pictured here. But take another look! It's one of those deceptive first impressions, as a second glance should confirm.

Take the angles of attack for example. Because of the downwash problem discussed so tediously elsewhere, we discovered that tail sections of conventional aircraft are always tilted down a bit. Helps keep things on the level. And when Alan Adler first filed his Skyro patent, with its "reverse angle" design, it looked as if, aerodynamically at least, he was blazing a new trail.

It turned out though that designers for the Caproni Aircraft Corporation anticipated a similar concept in the early 1920's when they drew up the plans for their amazing 9-wing, no tail seaplane,

a plane whose rearmost wings were mounted at a slight, but revolutionary, upward tilt. Nor did this fact go unnoticed by the patent examiners who held up approval for the Skyro application until they had been satisfied that claims for the two pieces of flying apparatus did not in fact overlap. As it turned out, there were structural differences and Adler's patent application was finally approved.

And in answer to your question, it crashed on its maiden flight.

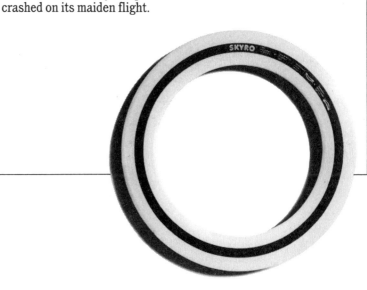

There followed a frustrating period of trial and error, encouraged by the computer findings but, thwarted by the fact that low-speed airfoil research is a widely neglected field, Adler was forced, more or less, to find his own way.

The breakthrough finally came in the course of prototyping a set of rings with small spoiler lips on the outside edge. The lip design struck the critical balance point: Flying forward, the rimmed airfoil is more sensitive to changes in its angle of attack than it is flying backward. But more important, it is precisely the *right* degree more sensitive.

It was a finely balanced aerodynamic tightrope act, made all the more impressive by the fact that the operating conditions were always changing—the "rope" wasn't being held very well. Nevertheless, the new design flew steadily over the whole range of possible speeds. It was a Skyro with an auto-pilot.

There followed all the usual problems inherent in translating prototype into production. Final changes in the airfoil and lip shape … mold design … finding the right combination of plastic and rubber …

It wasn't until late fall, 1984, that the first production Aerobie rolled off the line and flew, to everyone's instant relief, as well as the original prototypes.

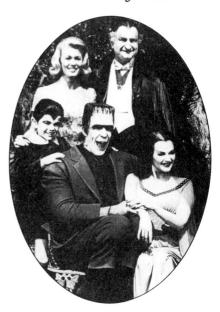

Challenge No. 10
The Family Plan

Organize the whole family. In order to count, it has *to be everybody* you can get a hold of. Drag them out to your throwing field. Everybody gets three chances for distance. *In order to count, the throw has to be caught.* Total everybody's best effort, take a family portrait, and send it in. We'll do a little handicapping here based on a secret formula involving a number of arcane things like hair color, age, horoscope, size of family, etc. Then we'll come up with a score and print the best three. *Hint:* Grandparents count double.

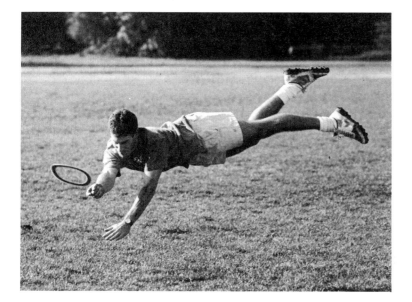

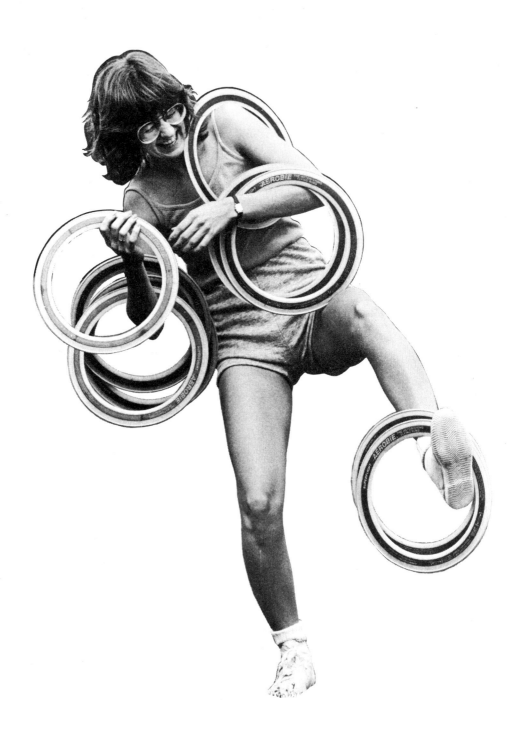

And Lastly, The Best Thing of All About the Aerobie®

In the course of this book, much has been made of the fact that an Aerobie is a revved up, high octane piece of flying apparatus and, in the hands of an experienced thrower, capable of leaping long fields in a single bound. What has been neglected though is something more important, because an Aerobie is also an incredibly low-frustration piece of remedial sporting equipment. It has brought a quality game of catch within the reach of *everyone*.

People with years of Frisbee failures behind them will suddenly find themselves throwing Aerobies over the startled heads of previously condescending friends, neighbors and spouses. And what's more, they'll be able to catch it on its return, via the "ringer" technique, no matter how ham-handed. The overall effect is magical. The same as a sudden leap into athletic stardom.

Downright intoxicating for a lifelong sports klutz.

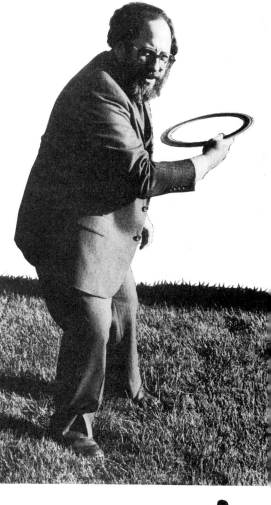

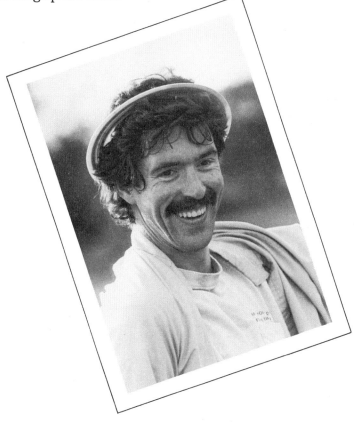

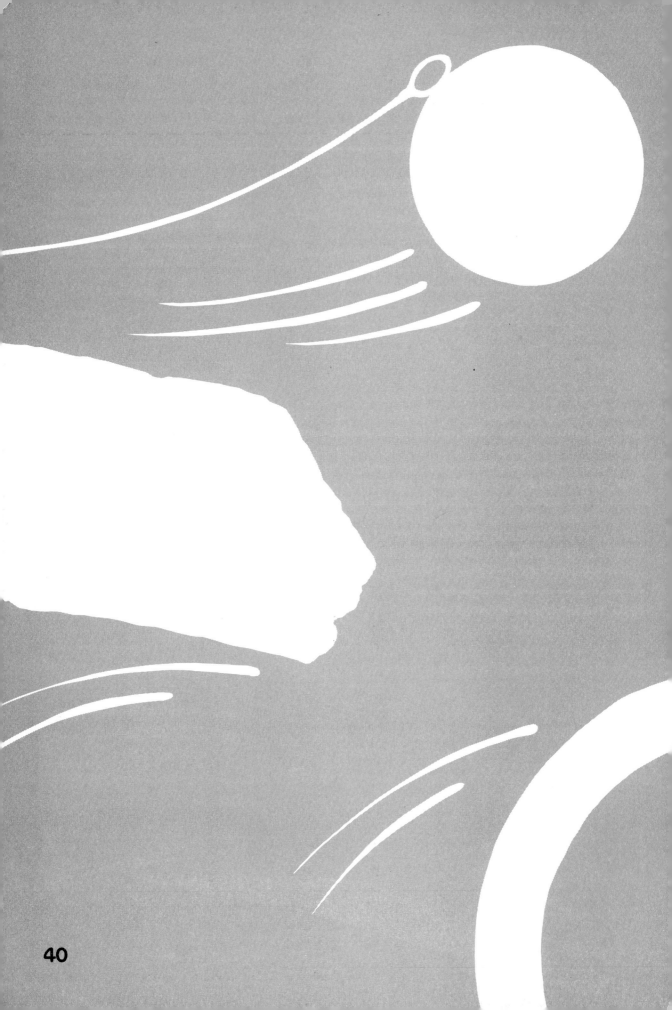

Appendices

I. The *Official* How-Far-Has-It-Been-Thrown Chart

Category A. Unaerodynamic Stuff

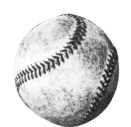

1. Baseball. 445 feet 10 inches

Glenn Gorbous on Aug. 1, 1957.

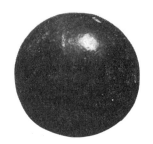

2. 16 lb. shotput. 72 feet 10¾ inches

Udo Beyer on June 25, 1983, in Los Angeles. The shotput sets a kind of standard for terrible aerodynamics.

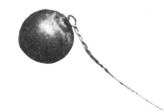

3. Hammer. 283 feet 3 inches

Yuri Sedykh on July 4, 1984, in Cork, Ireland.

4. Tree. 54 feet

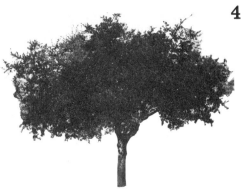

George Clark, in 1951 at the Scottish Highland Games. In Scotland, tree throwing is quite popular. It's called tossing the caber and, to be perfectly honest, the object is not specifically distance, but to flip the thing end for end. Obviously, which tree one chooses has a lot to do with one's success rate. The tree in question here was 120 pounds and 19 feet tall. Smallish for a tree perhaps, but an awesome piece of track and field equipment.

5. Brick. 146 feet 1 inch

Geoffrey Capes on July 19, 1978 at the Braybrook School, Cambridgeshire, England.

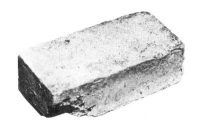

6. Javelin. 343 feet 10 inches.

Uwe Hohn on July 20, 1984, in East Berlin.

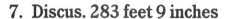

7. Discus. 283 feet 9 inches

Yuri Dumchev on May 29, 1983, in Moscow. Despite appearances, the discus has only slightly better aerodynamics than a brick.

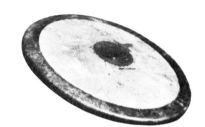

8. Beachball. 45 feet 6¾ inches

John Cassidy, April 30, 1985, in Palo Alto, California. (Anyone who has problems with this record, write your own book.)

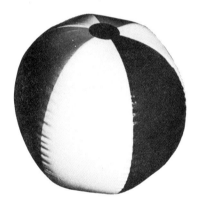

Overhead view of these records on a football field

baseball	
shotput	
hammer	
tree	
brick	
javelin	
discus	
beachball	

I. The *Official* How-Far-Has-It-Been-Thrown Chart

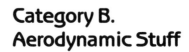

Category B. Aerodynamic Stuff

1. Boomerang. 750 feet (out and back, with a catch)

Peter Ruhf on June 28, 1982. Ruhf is an American who, in an insult-to-injury turnaround, set this record in Sydney, Australia.

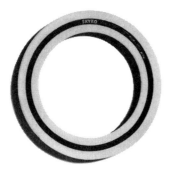

2. Skyro. 857 feet 8 inches

Tom McRann, June 9, 1980, at Golden Gate Park, San Francisco. The Skyro is Alan Adler's Aerobie prototype. It was his first marketed flying ring design, slightly smaller in diameter than the Aerobie and without the all-important stabilizing lip.

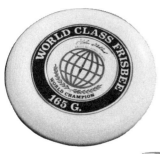

3. Frisbee.® 550 feet

Frank Aquilera on February 4, 1984. (There are no wind restrictions in the world of outdoor Frisbee records. This record was set with a following wind of indeterminate speed in Las Vegas, Nevada.)

boomerang
Skyro®
Frisbee®
paper airplane
Aerobie®
card

40

4. Aerobie.®

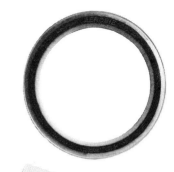

13″—1,257 feet. Scott Zimmerman on July 8, 1986, at Fort Funston, San Francisco, California.
10″—693 feet. Scott Zimmerman on November 4, 1987, at Sunset-Collier Park, San Diego, California.

5. Playing card. 185 feet 1 inch

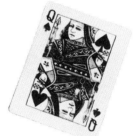

Kevin St. Onge on June 12, 1979, on the campus of the Henry Ford Community College, Dearborn, Michigan.

6. Paper airplane. 200 feet plus

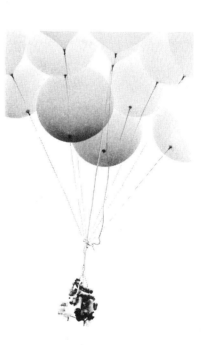

Designed by Alan Adler, thrown in the course of the Second Great Paper Airplane Contest in Seattle, Washington June 4, 1985. *Note:* The winning design was a paper version of the Aerobie, and the judges were so befuddled by (a) its extraordinary performance and (b) its circular shape, that they disqualified it and awarded the prize to a dart shaped design which flew only 144 feet. The subsequent uproar has become known as the Great Paper Airplane Controversy. Plans for building both planes (the winner and "the winner") are located in the appendix *Paper Flight.*

7. Lawnchair. 42 miles.

Larry Walters, San Pedro, California, July 3, 1982.*

*This record is unfortunately asterisked because Mr. Walters used helium balloons—42 of them to be exact. But the fact that he got high enough (16,000 feet) to pose an air traffic control problem plus the fact that he got back down by shooting out a few of his balloons with a BB gun, certainly renders the effort worthy of at least a footnote.

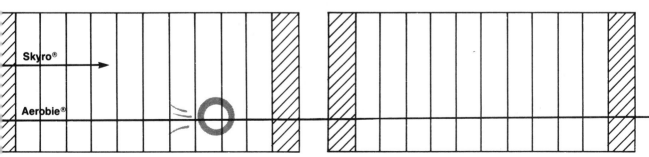

II. Paper Flight, and *The Great Paper Airplane Controversy*

After laboring for centuries in obscurity, serious paper airplane designers have had only two opportunities over the past 20 years to emerge into the light, and compete in the glare of world-wide publicity.

The First International Paper Airplane Contest was held in 1967 and sponsored by *Scientific American.* Thousands of small-scale aerodynamicists, accustomed to the relative privacy of movie theatre balconies and the back rows of high-school classrooms, were suddenly thrust onto the world's stage. It was a momentous event in aviation history.

The second tournament was held in 1985 and sponsored by the Smithsonian Museum and *Science 85,* and while the 1967 affair was relatively conflict free, the

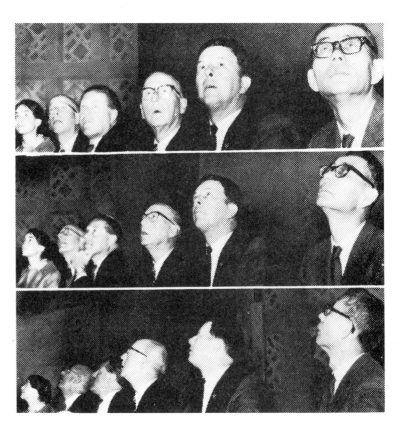

Figure 1. Jurors at the First International Paper Airplane Contest track one of the entries in the final elimination.

Second International Paper Airplane Contest became host to a dispute that has entered the annals of paper airplaning as *The Great Paper Airplane Controversy.*

The seeds of the conflict were sown when Alan Adler decided to enter with a paper Aerobie, and despite the fact that innovation was specifically encouraged in the tournament literature, called ahead to see if such a circular design would be acceptable.

It was, he was told, and thus approved, he went ahead and built what soon became the longest flying paper airplane in history, beating the second place finisher by more than 60 feet in the final fly-offs.

What followed was an unprecedented official reversal. Faced with the unquestioned superiority of the Aerobie design, the panel of judges suddenly disallowed it and promoted a dart-shaped design into first place.

The official explanation was that a round shape was not a *bona fide* paper airplane, plunging the debate straight to the heart of the paper airplane metaphysic.

Aerobie supporters argued, with simple, heartfelt logic, that (a) it's paper and (b) it flies.

Q.E.D.

Traditional paper airplane designers denounced this definition, declaring it to be "simplistic," "disingenuous," and "a vile trampling of the paper airplane 'aesthetic.'"

Given the depth of feelings involved, the issue is not likely to be settled in these pages. Therefore, lacking a clear mandate, both designs are included. The question of legitimacy is left as an exercise.

Paper Aerobie Blueprints and Instructions

1. You'll need a nice flat sheet of corrugated cardboard, about 10 inches square. The kind they put under take-out pizza is perfect. (*"Hi. We'd like an extra-large delivered to 1400 Belmont Drive. You can hold the pizza, but if you can bring along an extra piece of cardboard…"*).

2. Draw three circles on it. One with a radius of 5″, the second with a radius of 4⅞″, and the smallest with a radius of 3½″. On the right side of the page is a strip you can cut out and use as a compass for this part of the project. The correct distances are indicated on it.

5″
4⅞″

3½″

punch a pencil point through here

An Aerobie Building Paper Compass

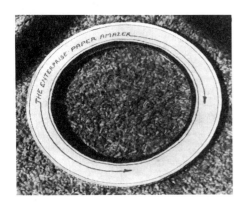

3. Cut along the outside and inside circles with some kind of sharp knife, an X-acto for example. Don't cut along the 4⅞″ circle, we'll use that later as a guide.

4. If you look closely, you'll see that you now have a cardboard ring. Try to fly it and you'll find it curving off to the left. That's because we're not done yet.

5. Flip a coin and determine which side of your ring is going to be the top. Then bend the *inside* of the ring up a bit. Work your way around the ring and go very slowly. The idea is to make the inside of the ring very slightly higher than the outside.

You can see if you've overdone it by tossing the ring and watching the way it curves. If it goes right, you've bent too much. Left, not enough. (Don't forget, lefties, reverse this stuff.)

Ideally, it should fly straight nearly all the way to the ground, when it will finally curve left.

At this point, you've got a good flier. Not a great one though. That doesn't come until you've created the spoiler lip.

6. Using a small knife, cut into the outer edge about ⅛″ deep, all the way around. This allows you to splay the edge out, making a spoiler lip, both top and bottom, about ⅛″ high, all the way around the ring. This is where the penciled-in circle at 4⅞″ comes in. It marks the inner limit to the spoiler lip.

7. Now for the final tuning. Head for the living room testing grounds. If it curves left, splay the *bottom* edge down more. If it flew right, splay the outer top edge *up* more.

When you're zeroed in, it will fly dead level and straight right down to the ground.

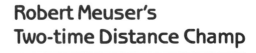

Robert Meuser's
Two-time Distance Champ

In the world of big-time paper airplaning, the name Robert Meuser is not one to be taken lightly. In 1967, the Berkeley physicist garnered first prize in the First International Paper Airplane Contest in the category of distance/non-professional. The event was sponsored by *Scientific American* and drew almost 12,000 entries.

Assembly Destructions

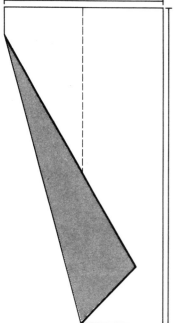
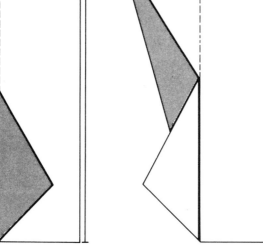
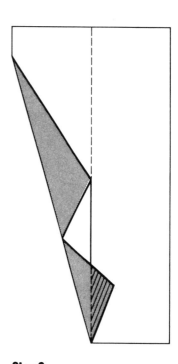

Step 1.

Step 2.

Step 3.

Cut the cross-hatched area off and
repeat Steps 1, 2 and 3.

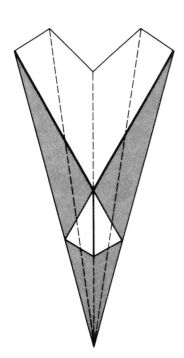
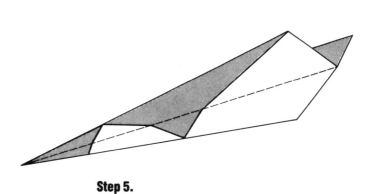

Step 4.

Cut the tail as illustrated,
fold along the center and glue.

Step 5.

You're ready. Wait 'til the teacher
turns around.

49

Books Available from Klutz

The Aerobie Book   The Bedtime Book
The Book of Classic Board Games
Boondoggle: A Book of Lanyard & Lacing
Braids & Bows   The Buck Book   Cat's Cradle
Country and Blues Guitar for the Musically Hopeless
Country and Blues Harmonica for the Musically Hopeless
Draw the Marvel™ Super Heroes™
Earthsearch: A Kids' Geography Museum in a Book
Everybody's Everywhere Backyard Bird Book
Explorabook: A Kids' Science Museum in a Book
Face Painting   The Foxtail® Book   The Hacky Sack Book
Hair: A Book of Styles and Braiding   The Incredible Clay Book
Juggling for the Complete Klutz
KidsCooking: A Very Slightly Messy Manual
KidsGardening: A Kid's Guide to Messing Around in the Dirt
KidsShenanigans: Great Things to Do That Mom and Dad Will Just
Barely Approve Of
KidsSongs   KidsSongs 2   KidsSongs Jubilee
KidsSongs Sleepyheads
KidsTravel: A Backseat Survival Kit
The Klutz Book of Card Games: For Sharks and Others
The Klutz Book of Jacks   The Klutz Book of Knots
The Klutz Book of Magic   The Klutz Book of Magnetic Magic
The Klutz Book of Marbles   The Klutz Yo-Yo Book
Make Believe: A Book of Costume and Fantasy
The Official Koosh Book   The Official Icky Poo Book
Pickup Sticks
Stop the Watch: A Book of Everyday Olympics
Table Top Football   The Time Book
The Unbelievable Bubble Book
Watercolor for the Artistically Undiscovered

FREE 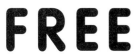 CATALOGUE!

(but there's a catch)

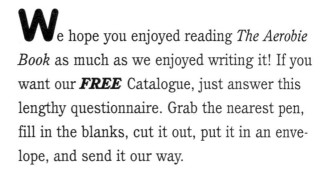

We hope you enjoyed reading *The Aerobie Book* as much as we enjoyed writing it! If you want our **FREE** Catalogue, just answer this lengthy questionnaire. Grab the nearest pen, fill in the blanks, cut it out, put it in an envelope, and send it our way.

KLUTZ.

2121 Staunton Court
Palo Alto, CA 94306

(or FAX us a copy at 1-800-524-4075)

Who Are You?   (You wonderful person you.)

❏ Kid   ❏ Grown-up   ❏ Somewhere in between   ❏ Girl   ❏ Boy

Name _____

Address _____

Telephone # _____

True or False!

T   F

❏   ❏   Someone gave me this book as a gift because they like me a whole lot!

❏   ❏   I bought this book for myself because I deserve it!

❏   ❏   This is the first **KLUTZ.** book I've ever bought.

A Personal Question!

I'm the kind of person who spends this kind of money on a gift for a friend:

❏ Less than $10   ❏ $10-15   ❏ $15-20   ❏ $20-25

❏ For the right gift, whatever it's worth!

My Bright Ideas!

Tell us what you thought about this book... _____

Complaints here. ❏ (please don't go outside the box)

Consider the Following:

The strongest quarterbacks in the NFL today can throw a football the full length of the field, 300 feet. With a baseball, the best professionals can cover quite a bit more, about 500 feet on the fly. Meanwhile, the world's record for the javelin is 343 feet. These are all incredible throws, near the limit of human abilities...

But a good 16 year old could beat any of them with an Aerobie.

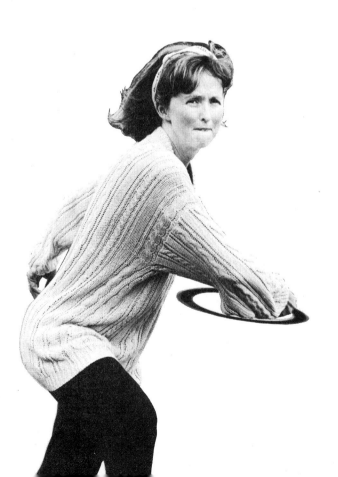